The Simple Guide to Clinical Hiring

The Simple Guide to Clinical Hiring

PENNY M. CROW
M. CHRISTINE KALISH
SHARON Z. GINCHANSKY

MGMA
Medical Group Management Association®

Item: 1021

ISBN: 978-1-56829-683-8

Printed in the United States of America

10 9 8 7 6 5 4 3 2 1

Contents

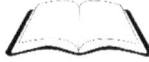

Purpose of the Hiring Guide

"People are not your most important asset. The right people are." – Jim Collins

The Basics

This book will help you think about hiring in ways you haven't thought about it before. Throughout this book, you will see small icons that will indicate three categories of information.:

	General information that is repeated in each of the hiring guides published by MGMA
	Specific information that is required information for the category of jobs being discussed and is only in this manual.
	These are isolated boxes meant to highlight information like pro tips and best practices.
	Key takeaway summaries are included throughout.

The core information in this guide is focused on the full recruitment cycle, outlined below:

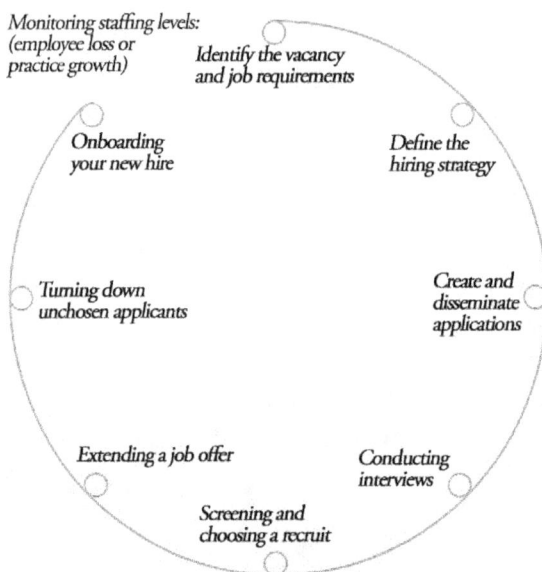

Monitoring staffing levels: (employee loss or practice growth)

Identify the vacancy and job requirements

Onboarding your new hire

Define the hiring strategy

Turning down unchosen applicants

Create and disseminate applications

Extending a job offer

Conducting interviews

Screening and choosing a recruit

Why does a medical practice need a hiring guide?

For many practices, hiring and recruitment is not a full-time, or even regular, activity. This hiring guide is written for everyone who manages staff or might be responsible for tasks involving human resources. This can be a narrow or broad group of resources and can include practice managers, physician-owners, and other staff, such as supervisors, recruiters, interviewers, trainers, compensation managers, HR specialists, legal/compliance coordinators, and researchers.

This guide takes the reader through the entire process from job analysis to description creation and through to hiring and onboarding. While it includes documents, tools, and related job descriptions, the guide is written in such a way that a practice can reference a certain section to focus in on just that information. This manual is tactical and process-oriented, providing step by step instructions for hiring tasks that might not be included in the daily workstream. It outlines the proactive strategies required to define, attract, and retain qualified applicants.

One of the challenges in a medical practice, especially smaller ones with limited resources, is the limited preparation before a vacancy occurs. When the manager receives a two-week notice from someone considered to be a valued or key employee, a couple of things tend to occur. First, the manager thinks they have more time than really exists to replace that employee; second, the manager imagines they might be able to convince the employee to stay. The reality is that the manager must act, and act quickly. Without a clear-cut process that can be immediately executied to begin the recruitment process, the gap for the practice may have nearly-immediate impacts on day-to-day operations. This manual, when used to its maximum benefit, will assist the medical practice in building a base for recruiting, hiring, and retaining staff that will allow the responsiveness and quick pivots required for today's medical practice environment.

This guide addresses the consistent processes and points out those that are specific to the job category in the title. While the rules and regulations for hiring and recruiting may be similar, different job levels and categories present unique challenges along the way. This tool provides tricks, tips, and best-practice ideas to support every size medical organization.

All staff should have access to this tool. Too often, organizations limit human resources and hiring functions to those who supervise, manage, or own the practice. Almost all staff, at one time or another, will be asked to participate in some part of the recruitment and hiring process. This guide also ensures *everyone* follows the appropriate process when bringing new staff into the practice. Additionally, this guide may help employees understand how their job relates to others in the practice. Sharing this information, so employees understand cause and effect, job performance, and the importance of improvement, benefits the entire organization.

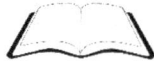

Analyzing Medical Practice Staffing

"Time spent on hiring is time well spent." – Robert Half

As much as an organization wants to think that they are proactive about planning for staff changes, too often those plans are set aside when faced with the clear priority to provide excellent care to patients and deliver the associated day-to-day tasks. When a vacancy opens within an organization, the natural inclination is to move forward with filling the position as quickly as possible. The better strategy is to use the vacancy as an opportunity to assess staffing needs and determine if the organization can benefit from doing more than just hiring for the same job. This activity will take more time, but what the practice will gain in the long run by having a well-rounded team cannot be underestimated.

Even before the practice writes or updates a job description, the manager needs to make sure the projected position will meet the needs of the organization. Asking some questions and completing a short analysis will set the baseline for the hiring process and define an order of operations.

The first step is to better understand why there is an opening. What caused the individual to leave the position?

Reasons can include:

- Workload
  - o Real or perceived workload disparities will create disagreements in the practice.
- Personality and fit
  - o Company culture can make or break a team, and team attitude can make or break the culture.
- Managerial issues
  - o People don't leave jobs; they leave managers.
- Compensation
  - o Real or perceived compensation discrepancies create disgruntled employees.
- Training
  - o A practice cannot expect the best from employees if they aren't trained appropriately.
- Personal
  - o Life events and family commitments that are out of the practice's control.
- Career Advancement
  - o It is difficult to provide numerous advancement opportunities in a smaller practice, however, there are different methods of addressing that in order to retain employees.

The practice can determine the answer to these questions through employee interviews and exit interviews—and through observing workflow and the personal interactions. There are tools available to model the process. The key is to keep this simple.

Depending on the answer to the above question, focus on different analyses to determine reasonable changes. Realistically, some things cannot be changed, but the practice may be able to balance that out with the issues that can be changed. For example, if this is about workload, analyze the staffing changes that can be made so the workloads can be distributed more equally and effectively. Small practices are challenged because staff may fill several roles. Roles can grow organically because a staff member may be a stellar performer and won't say no to the extra workload. This easily occurs when services are added that only require a few hours a week, such as scheduling for a part-time provider. The challenge is that workload can grow exponentially and eventually become unmanageable, creating employee dissatisfaction.

Job analysis is usually designed to be work-oriented or worker-oriented. A *work-oriented analysis* results in specific tasks being identified in a typical workday. For example, the receptionist in a small practice may answer phones, schedule appointments, collect monies, and balance the cash drawer. An example of a work-oriented result would be: 'It's time to convert to an electronic process rather than doing a task manually.' A *worker-oriented analysis* focuses on the qualities of the employee, such as knowledge, skills, abilities, and other characteristics (KSAOs) that will contribute to an employee's success in the job.

> A *work-oriented analysis* results in specific tasks being identified in a typical workday. A *worker-oriented analysis* consists of identifying the knowledge, skills, abilities, and other personal attributes that will be important to your practice. It is easier to teach how to complete tasks than it is to make someone fit your culture. Knowing exactly what is needed in a person will make it clearer to identify and hire toward.

Although it is important to hire competent staff, it is equally important that the competent staff also have emotional intelligence, empathy, communication, and other soft skills. This guide discusses how to identify these skills through interviewing techniques. Making poor hiring decisions costs money, creates liability, and results in lost time. Using best practices mitigates these risks. For example, the receptionist needs to be friendly, detail-oriented, reliable, and trustworthy. Whatever job analysis format you use,make sure you are consistent when writing all job descriptions. This information can also be used to determine the salary for a position, training needs, and the performance management process for feedback and evaluation.

Reviewing Relevant Regulations

Before getting into the specifics of the job, it is important to be aware of employment laws that may affect your individual positions. The section below is taken from MGMA's *Job Description Manual for Medical Practices*, 4th Edition (2019).

FLSA (1938)

The **Fair Labor Standards Act of 1938 (FLSA)**, as amended, established minimum wages, equal pay, and overtime; outlawed child labor; and specified record-keeping affecting most full- and part-time employees. One critical part of the law spotlighted in job descriptions is the designation of "exempt" or "nonexempt" job classifications. *Exempt* means that employees holding these jobs are not eligible for overtime pay. These are primarily professional positions. For example, if registered by the state, nurses meet the learned professional exemption and may be classified as exempt if paid on a salary basis of at least $455 per week. Nonexempt employees, such as clerks, are eligible for overtime when they work more than 12 hours in a workday or if they work more than 40 hours in a workweek. The Department of Labor designates which jobs are in which category. The designations do change occasionally. Supervisors should work with an HR specialist to make sure they know which positions are exempt or nonexempt and what that means in terms of overtime pay and other factors.

EPA (1963)

The **Equal Pay Act of 1963 (EPA)** applies to all employers covered by the federal wage and hour law under the Fair Labor Standards Act (see below). It requires that men and women be given equal pay for equal work in the same establishment. The job content, as described in the job description, determines whether jobs are substantially equal.

OSH Act (1970)

The **Occupational Safety and Health Act of 1970 (OSH Act)** established regulations to provide for the health and safety of employees on the job and the Occupational Safety and Health Administration (OSHA). The Act aims to ensure better working conditions by establishing guidelines for employers and employees on work environment conditions. The section in a job description titled "work environment" is a response to this Act and must consider such environmental factors as lighting, workspace, and identifying hazards. Employers must document, track, and report occupational injury and illness trends. Every medical practice should have a safety training plan and conduct such training during orientation and at regular times during employment. Examples of training include courses on body mechanics, infection control, and biohazard protection.

EEO (1972)

The **Equal Employment Opportunity Act of 1972**, referred to as **EEO**, extends the anti-discrimination provisions of Title VII of the 1964 Civil Rights Act. Your lawyer and an HR specialist can help ensure your job descriptions, hiring, and other employment practices comply with the mandate that individuals must be protected against employment discrimination on the basis of race, color, sex, national origin, and religion. It applies to employers with fifteen or more employees. There are two other legal issues to consider. When writing job descriptions, list only the minimum necessary requirements such as education and experience. It is acceptable to note preferred or desirable additional factors, but the emphasis must be on those that are necessary to ensure members of minority groups are not artificially screened out. Also, job descriptions should not state that a job can only be performed by a licensed professional when that is not actually a requirement of the state. For example, states require RNs to be licensed; however, medical assistants are not required to be licensed.

ADA (1990)

The **Americans with Disabilities Act of 1990 (ADA)** prohibits private employers, state and local governments, employment agencies, and labor unions from discriminating against qualified individuals with disabilities in job application procedures, hiring, firing, advancement, compensation, job training, and other aspects of employment. The ADA covers employers with fifteen or more employees. The Act does not protect every disabled person. The person also must be qualified, i.e., an individual who, with or without reasonable accommodation, can perform the essential functions of the job in question. The job description must clearly define those essential job responsibilities, the work environment, the equipment operated, the physical demands, as well as the required knowledge, skills, and abilities. Any person can then be compared with this job profile to ensure the qualification standard is met. HR specialists have the expertise to ensure that you comply with this critical legal regulation.

HIPAA (1996)

The **Health Insurance Portability and Accountability Act of 1996 (HIPAA)** not only focuses on accountability for ensuring patient privacy and confidentiality, it also protects the ability to continue to qualify for health insurance benefits if the employee changes or loses his or her job. It is the patient privacy and confidentiality piece that impacts a job description. Although job descriptions do not need to specify the "need-to-know" level of a job, they frequently emphasize the confidentiality requirement. In all cases, it is important for the supervisor to clearly define a job's confidentiality factors. For example, a clinician caring for a patient needs to know the person's diagnosis; a janitor in the facility does not.

HITECH (2009)

The **Health Information Technology for Economic and Clinical Health Act of 2009 (HITECH)** provides HHS with the authority to establish programs to improve healthcare quality, safety, and efficiency through the promotion of health IT, including electronic health records and private and secure electronic health information exchange. HITECH greatly impacts the need for technological proficiency.

Much of the listed legislation and regulation will affect the medical practice in some way.

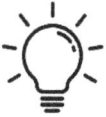

> **Pro Tip:** Keeping your eyes on the prize.
>
> - Determine what skillsets can be taught and what must be brought to the table.
> - Document the required skillsets.
> - Determine traits.
> - Determine what is the practice's responsibility to teach, remembering that training is not a one and done.
> - Expand the touchpoints for finding competent candidates; this will help you resist the impulse to make the easy hire.
> - Be aware that quickly-achieved, short-term relief will almost always equal long-term aggravation.
> - Don't forget that it will tend to cost the practice from 3 to 5 times the annual salary if the hire is a mistake.

Conducting a Job Analysis

In larger practices, a consultant may be contracted to complete a job analysis. However, it isn't necessary to bring someone from the outside. The internal hiring manager can use the same tips and tricks for success. First, interview leadership to determine what expectations were set for the job. Next, interview the supervisor of that position, and then, finally, interview the person that actually does the job. It is always educational to see the disconnect between the three descriptions for the same position. This sort of job analysis can help address these discrepancies and provide a decision tool for what the roles and responsibilities of each job should be and, thereby, create a performance standard.

Another way to conduct a job analysis is to observe the current holder of the position and document the tasks being performed. Observing rather than interviewing allows a practice leader to determine if each of these tasks and processes are necessary for today's medical practice. Alternatively, some practices find it useful to have employees complete preprinted questionnaires. And last, but not least, other resources from MGMA may be appropriate for determining the specific tasks and KSAOs necessary for a job. It is important to document all essential functions of the job within the job description. Essential functions are what are considered when an employee requires accommodations made under the ADA. Questions to determine essential job functions include:

- Is this task truly necessary for the job?
- How often does this task have to be done?
- What percentage of time is spent doing this task?
- What happens if the employee doesn't do this task? (Are there consequences?)
- Can the tasks be done differently?
- Can the task be reassigned to someone else?

Now is the time to consider exactly what tasks the position is performing for the team and ask if those tasks:

- are necessary;
- add value; and
- support the core business, which is taking care of the patient.

In addition, consider if technology can be implemented or updated to relieve manual processes. You may find that the position is not really what you thought it was, and so making modifications may ensure retention in that position for the next candidate while boosting the productivity of the entire area or practice. Broken processes and incorrect staffing create significant inefficiencies and cost the practice in quality service, decreasing both patient and employee satisfaction.

If compensation is an issue, first look at the salary or hourly wage relative to the market. Market survey data is available through many sources to determine if the position is being compensated fairly for the work expected. Often this data is difficult to find, particularly when positions are identified differently by each practice. The front desk staff could be patient services representatives or medical receptionist, both doing the same job. When this happens, more analysis is required. Always look in your own backyard to determine if certain positions tend to move frequently, then consider other benefits to encourage retention. In all cases, re-evaluate the budget to see if there is room to increase the salary to be competitive and attract top candidates. Remember that a change for one equals a change for all. Adjusting compensation to keep one employee is never a good idea for the organization.

Take the time to step back and assess workflows to make sure the organizational structure is producing the optimal results. Ask yourself these questions:

- Are there inefficiencies that can be addressed?
- Are there processes that are broken?
- Are there reasons for all tasks being performed?

An individual new to the practice is not accustomed to doing things the usual way, so there is a great opportunity to map out process improvements that can be put into place with a fresh perspective.

Then, always consider personality and fit. Organizational culture, whether the practice is large or small, dictates employee and consequently, patient satisfaction. Be able to understand and communicate the company culture. Know if it's important to have a voice. That will help plan and focus your search. Know who and what you are hiring for.

Wrapping up: Analyzing Medical Practice Staffing

Taking the time to do a thorough analysis of your medical practice staffing is well worth the investment. Before leaping in to quickly replace a departing employee, make sure to gather all the information required to determine the correct staffing solution going forward for the practice. It is also imperative to make sure you understand the market for the role you do wish to hire and that your compensation package is competitive to acquire the quality staff the practice requires.

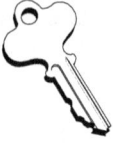

Key Takeaways

- Reconsider simply recycling the same job description to fill a new vacancy.

- Assess the reasons for the vacancy and make modifications as necessary to make the role as successful as possible.

- Go a step further and see if there are changes that can be made to current processes and workflows to make the organization perform at a higher level.

- Clearly understand your practice culture

Clinical Roles
within the Medical Practice

You can have the best strategy and the best building in the
world, but if you don't have the hearts and minds of the people
who work with you, none of it comes to life."—Renee West

There are key market drivers that are creating challenges for medical
practices. These include a changing regulatory environment,
reimbursement challenges, larger consumer payments with decreasing
margins for medical practices, and patients recognizing that they
have a voice in their care. Additionally, social media provides instant
information and opinions about the provision of healthcare.

The American Medical Association (AMA) has identified empathy
and communication as the two necessary soft skills in today's healthcare
environment. Patients expect more from their clinical providers. These
high expectations impact the medical practice at almost every entry
and care point. This hiring manual focuses on the clinical group of job
descriptions. Regardless of the size of the practice, the clinical team is
the primary point for patient care. Clinical jobs within a practice may
include the nursing staff, therapists, technicians, and providers. In order
to create and expand access for the patients of the medical practice,
the clinical providers are teaming in more integrative ways. This poses
different hiring and recruiting challenges for more forwarding thinking
practices.

The job descriptions in this category may include:

- Practice Nurse
- Medical Assistant
- Therapist
- Technician
- Physician

Care providers are expected to:

- Work directly with patients.
- Document medical history.
- Use and maintain medical equipment.
- Order and perform diagnostic tests.
- Observe vitals.
- Provide a prognosis based on the treatment progress.
- Listen with empathy.
- Give dedicated time to patients and family.
- Teach patients and caregivers.
- Teach peers, colleagues and subordinates.

Not everyone is cut out for direct patient care. Care providers are a combination of technical skill and heart. Recent surveys have shown that patients expect clinicians to be open with communication, responsive to questions, and competent. It is often the bedside manner that can determine the relationship outcomes between patient and provider. It is human nature to tolerate mistakes when the provider is more likeable, open, and personable. Staff fulfill different roles and may crossover those roles, depending on the needs of the practice. This guide focuses on the recruitment, hiring, and retention process for these key positions.

As a group, these positions, require the following skills:

- Have sound clinical decision-making skills,
- Be able to ask significant questions,

- Listen well,
- Be empathetic,
- Be observant,
- Communicate effectively, and
- Simplify complex issues for better understanding.

Let's break down this category into groups and consider their essential functions with the related characteristics that will make a potential candidate successful in that job function.

Practice Nurse

There are some clinics that will only hire registered or licensed practical nurses. Those tend to be specialty practices with complicated patients and in-office procedures. The responsibilities and skills needed for practice nurses include:

- Complete patient assessments.
- Document objective and subjective data.
- Assist physicians and other providers.
- Manage medication reconciliation.
- Operate medical equipment.
- Handle patient phone communications.
- Have a robust understanding of HIPAA, OSHA and CLIA guidelines.,
- Perform injections and venipunctures.

Degrees, certification, and licenses required can include:

- Degrees requirements differ by state.
- Registered Nurse (RN), Nurse Practitioner (NP), or Advanced Practice Registered Nurse (APRN),
- Many certifications are available for nurses, including Clinical Nurse Leader (CLE), Certified Nurse Educator (CNE), and Trauma Certified Registered Nurse (TCRN).
- Current state board of nursing licensing
- Communication

Their competencies will include:

- Customer/client focus,
- Teamwork orientation,
- Problem solving and analysis,
- Communication proficiency
- Learning orientation,
- Ethical standards and conduct,
- Stress management skills,
- Composure, and
- Discretion.

Some of the success characteristics include:

- Balance proactive and reactive problem-solving skills,
- Attention to detail,
- Excellent communication skills ,
- Scientific thinker, and
- Patient education skills.

A successful nurse will understand how to bridge the gap between the technical verbiage, medical business, and the people component. Nurses need numerical reasoning as well as being able to complete basic math calculations. It may be necessary for the nurse to take complex messages and convert them to useful communications to the patient and family. Earning a license does not always equate to these success factors. A practice must carefully assess and question for these characteristics and skills. It is easier to find the best-fit nurse candidates when you know exactly for what the requirements are for your practice. There is no reason to hire and pay for more than is needed for the job. Qualified nurses know that they must be flexible in their expectation of the day, the tasks, and the outcomes.

Medical Assistant

Although all states allow medical assistants, it is important to know the applicable state laws regarding the scope of service. For example, some states do not allow medical assistants to do venipunctures.

Medical assistants are usually trained to assist in both the front office and clinical area.

Responsibilities and skills for medical assistants could include:

- Obtain basic health history from patient.
- Administer medications.
- Provide basic patient education.
- Schedule appointments.

Degrees, certification, and licenses required can include:

- College degrees are not required for medical assistants.
- Many certifications are available for medical assistants, including Certified Medical Assistant (CMA), Registered Medical Assistant (RMA), and National Certified Medical Assistant (NCMA).
- There are also specialty certifications available for medical assistants.

Their competencies include:

- Empathetic listener,
- Outgoing,
- Able to follow direction,
- Organized, and
- Problem solver.

Some of the success characteristics for medical assistants include:

- Excellent verbal and written communication skills;
- Strong interpersonal, organizational, and customer service skills;
- Attention to detail; and
- Initiative.

One size does not fit all with medical assistants. Training for this position can differ significantly from program to program, so experience is frequently a key decision-making factor. The medical assistant may be the only care provider in the office in many practices. They must understand the scope of their training while still being open to learning and expanding their skills sets under the appropriate supervision of other care providers. For example, some practices require the medical assistant to assist the physician in simple procedures. It may be their responsibility to run some lab tests. Again, it is the education, experience, and legal limitations that will drive the specific scope for the medical assistant position. Most importantly, the medical assistant must be willing to ask for help and guidance when needed. The patient's safety must always be the number one priority of all care providers. The practice must determine the need prior to interviewing so that boundaries, if needed, are established from the start.

Therapist

Some practices may have onsite therapists for patient care. This could include a physical therapist, occupational therapist, respiratory therapist, or speech therapist, among others.

Responsibilities and skills for therapists could include:

- Possess up-to-date knowledge of treatment practices.
- Regularly update skills to learn new treatment techniques.
- Excellent interpersonal communication skills.
- Analytical and logical thinking.

Degrees, certification, and licenses required can include:

- It is important to know the state laws regarding licensure, certification, and scope of service for each specialty. Some specialties require more advanced formal education than others.
- Look to the specific professional association or governing board for more information.

Their competencies may include:

- Ability to solve problems independently.

- Knowledge of and compliance with state and federal regulatory requirements.
- Understand reimbursement guidelines per payer.
- Treat patients with different personalities and across all ages.

Some of the success characteristics include:

- Ability to communicate effectively both verbally and in writing,
- Compassionate,
- Attentive to details, and
- Scientific knowledge of modalities.

Aptitude test attributes given in colleges for therapists include assessing for self-motivation, time management, and flexibility. Being a good therapist goes beyond the scientific knowledge, but it is the therapist that may have significant influence on patient's treatment plans. Not only are the therapists care provider,s but many times they must have the personality to be a cheerleader for patients during challenging times.

Technicians

This group includes radiology techs, ultrasound techs, and medical technologists. Each state regulates education, certification, and licensure of healthcare technician specialties. A radiology tech has specific technical education using medical imaging equipment for diagnostic purposes. Ultrasound techs use a sonography machine that utilizes high-frequency sound waves to collect reflected echoes of organs and tissues. Medical technologists operate and maintain the lab equipment used to analyze specimens for diagnostic studies.

In each of the specialty fields, a physician will ultimately be the interpreter of the testing results. However, the physician relies heavily on the expertise of technicians.

Responsibilities and skills include

- Knowledgeable in their specialty.
- Attentive to their processes and equipment.
- Must be able understand the science behind their work.

Degrees, certification, and licenses required include:

- Generally require at least an Associate's degree.
- Certification and licensing determined by state law. Varies widely.

Competencies include:

- Effective in their use of specialized equipment.
- Be able to communicate with patients and other care providers regarding the processes and results.

Some of the success characteristics include:

- Detail oriented,
- Diligent and exacting,
- Strong interpersonal skills ,
- Excellent technical skills,,
- Comfortable taking responsibility for the safety and well-being of their patients

The radiology and ultrasound technicians will work closely with patients. However, a lab tech may be in solitude working mainly with specimens and equipment. All technicians will need to be detail oriented and attentive to the smallest changes. Although the tests will be run similarly and sometimes precisely the same as others, the day will be full of surprises as patients come and go. Technicians will need to easily adapt to the work pace.

Physicians

There is a significant shortage of physicians in the United States. Recruiting for physicians has become an HR specialty in itself. MGMA has many resources that discuss recruitment of physicians, compensation plans, RVUs, and building practices. Refer to these resources for more information. Suffice it to say, physicians also have their responsibilities and skills, competencies, and success characteristics.

Responsibilities and skills could include:

- Diagnose and treat medical conditions.
- Order lab tests and interpret the test results.
- Maintain confidentiality.
- Maintain impartiality.
- Explain procedures or prescribed treatments to patients.
- Document care in electronic medical record.
- Apply correct diagnostic and procedure codes.

Degrees, certification, and licenses required include:

- Medical degree,
- Completed U.S. Medical Licensing Examination
- Board certification
- Current state medical license,
- DEA license ,

Competencies include:

- Empathy and listening skills
- Excellent decision-making skills and communication

Success factors include:

- Organizational and time management skills
- Ability to make effective decisions
- Innate ability to manage change
- The willingness and ability to handle uncertainty and conflicting demands
- Remaining calm under pressure.

Several of the medical universities have taken a new approach for training physicians. Students may see patients from day one in medical school. Emotional intelligence is being integrated into the educational vocabulary. As patients have become more educated, they expect soft skills as well as knowledge from their physicians. Emotional intelligence requires self-awareness, empathy, compassion, and humility. These are not part of the traditional curriculum and culture inculcated in physicians.

Wrapping up: Clinical Roles

This chapter is a simplistic orientation to the clinical job category. A more thorough listing of clinical job descriptions is provided in Appendix A. Hiring practices should identify those candidates best qualified to serve in these positions. Care providers have the ability to create the overall patient access culture and experience. Hiring and retention practices must be targeted and specific to support the provision of care. In choosing candidates for clinical positions, it is important to identify in advance the skills and personality that will fit the position for the care of your patients. Now that you have a grasp on analyzing staffing and where clinical roles fit into the medical practice structure, the next chapter will walk through the steps to create a job description.

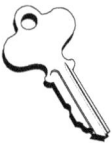

Key Takeaways

- Soft skills and emotional intelligence are key to successful employees in the clinical job category.
- These positions focus on delivering care while integrating the implications from federal, state, and local regulations.
- Continuing education to keep up with current knowledge and trends in their specialty is generally a requirement for these positions.

Preparing the Job Description

"Under conditions of complexity, not only are checklists a help, they are required for success." - Atul Gawande

Once the cause of the vacancy has been analyzed, it is necessary to determine if the job description is still valid. A job description is a necessary tool that explains how the tasks and duties of a specific job fit into the practice's overall mission and strategic goals. It is important to keep job descriptions up to date, but there is no better time to reassess a position than when it is, or is about to be, vacant.

Writing the Job Description

All job descriptions within the practice should look the same. Standardization and consistency are two of the best defenses in human resource management. Job description methodology continues to be the safest way for employers to have documentation that supports employment decisions and avoids legal issues and complications in hiring, training, and terminating staff. Most importantly, a job description's primary purpose remains stable: to clearly communicate how the employee helps fulfill the goals of the organization. One way to write a job description is to answer the following questions. These answers will design a best-practice-formatted job description. Below are the seventeen core questions to be answered about the position.

Below each question in a gray box is an illustrative (not comprehensive) example response.

1. What is the job title?

- Make the title reflect what the job does. Not only is it important for the employee to understand the title, but a patient reading a name tag needs to be able to determine what this person does. Keeping it simple is always the best naming convention, so be cautious about being creative with titles. Simplicity is one of the best communication tools for the employee and patients to understand the role.

> **Job title:** Office Manager

2. What is the job classification?

- The Fair Labor Standards (FLSA) is very specific regarding exempt vs. non-exempt positions. *Non-exempt* means that you must pay overtime. Conversely, an *exempt* role is one that is management- or leadership-focused and oversees other staff. Know your state laws and the legal requirements to determine if overtime will be paid on daily or weekly work hours over the standard eight-hour workday. Many practices want to save money by making all their clinical positions exempt to prevent overtime, but the level of responsibility is a primary consideration of job classification. When in doubt, consult an HR professional or attorney for clarification. This conservative approach will protect the practice and the employee from violating IRS rules.

> **Job classification:** Exempt

3. **To whom does this position report?**

- This should list the title of the person they will be their supervisor. Keep in mind that the CEO or owner may still report to a board of directors, partners, or investors.
- Dotted lines between multiple supervisors is not recommended.

> **Reports to:** Practice Owner

4. **When was the job description last reviewed?**

- It is helpful to make sure the job is still relevant by dating the job description, which can help trigger a re-assessment if enough time has passed. Nothing can hurt a new employee's satisfaction faster than having the wrong expectations for the job. It is particularly important for executive positions to determine the scope of work executive and the level of expertise needed from the very beginning.

> **Date:** 08.01.2019

5. **What is the summary of the overall job duties?**

- This is a summary that allows an employee or candidate to quickly know the expectations.

> **Summary:** A management position responsible for the daily operations of the medical practice.

6. **What are the essential job responsibilities for this position?**

- It is important from an employment law defense perspective that essential job responsibilities are listed to determine the applicability of ADA accommodations. The employee will need to be able to successfully complete these specific responsibilities with reasonable accommodations.

- These are the tasks that regardless of physical or mental ability must be done in this individual job.

Essential Job Responsibilities:

- Ensure compliance with current healthcare regulations, medical laws, federal and state laws, and high ethical standards.
- Oversee daily office operations and delegate authority to assigned supervisors.
- Assist supervisors in developing and implementing short- and long-term work plans and objectives for clerical functions.
- Develop guidelines for prioritizing work activities, evaluating effectiveness, and modifying activities as necessary. Ensure that office is staffed appropriately.
- Assist in the recruiting, hiring, orientation, development, and evaluation of clerical staff.
- Establish and maintain an efficient and responsive patient flow system.
- Oversee and approve office supply inventory, ensure that mail is opened and processed, and offices are opened and closed according to procedures.
- Support and uphold established practice policies, procedures, objectives, quality improvement, safety, environmental and infection control, and codes and requirements of accreditation and regulatory agencies.

7. **What are the competencies (KSAOs) needed?**

- It is important for the practice and potential candidate to assess if they are a good fit for each other. This is only possible if the competencies (KSAO) are identified in advance.

- Describe the personal attributes that this employee must have to be successful in this role.

Competencies:

Knowledge

- Knowledge of policies and procedures to manage operations and ensure effective patient care.
- Knowledge of the principles and practices of healthcare administration, fiscal management, and government regulationsand reimbursements.
- Knowledge of Electronic Health Systems.
- Knowledge of Practice Management Systems.
- Knowledge of medical practices, terminology, and reimbursement policies.
- This position requires strong working knowledge of managed care plans, insurance carriers, referrals, and precertification procedures.

Skills

- Skill in exercising a high degree of initiative, judgment, and discretion.
- Skill in analyzing situations accurately and taking effective action.
- Skill in establishing and maintaining effective working relationships.
- Skill in organizing work, delegating and achieving goals and objectives.
- Skill in exercising judgment and discretion in developing, interpreting, and implementing departmental policies and procedures.
- Mastery of spoken and written English.

- Additional languages preferred.
- Possess strong human relations, communication, problem solving, and organizational skills to interact with a variety of customers, payers, vendors, and personnel within and outside the institution.

Abilities:

- Ability to work under pressure, communicate, and present information.
- Ability to read, interpret, and apply clinic policies and procedures.
- Ability to identify problems, recommend solutions, and organize and analyze information.
- Ability to establish priorities and coordinate work activities.
- Ability to work independently and be goal-directed.
- Effectively multitask without compromising quality.
- Ability to comprehend and excel in both verbal and written communication, including proper telephone
- Ability to communicate with individuals and small groups with credibility and confidence.

Other:

- Willingness and desire to maintain regular and acceptable attendance; may be required to work weekend, holiday, or overtime hours.
- Willingness and drive to handle complex, difficult interactions, remain calm under stress, manage emotional situations, display empathy, and maintain positive communication within a rapidly changing/ dynamic environment.

8. **Are there any supervisory responsibilities?**

- Not all people are leaders and teachers. Supervisory responsibilities include both those attributes. The practice can protect itself by establishing supervision expectations from the beginning. Identify any direct reports.

> **Direct reports:** Business Office Manager, Facilities Manager, Administrative Assistant, Receptionist.

9. **What equipment is does the job require?**

   - Anything that may affect the employee's working conditions such as climate, noise, hours, construction.

   > **Equipment:** Employee expected to be able to use standard office equipment, including computers, fax machines, copiers, printers, telephones, etc.

10. **What is the work environment?**

    - Anything that may affect the employee's working conditions such as climate, noise, hours, construction.

    > **Work environment:** Employee works in a collaborative medical office environment with a private office for confidential conversations. Moderate noise (i.e. business office with computers, phone, and printers, light traffic). Ability to work in a confined area. Ability to sit at a computer terminal for an extended period of time.

11. **What are the physical and mental demands of the essential job functions?**

    - Identify any lifting, bending, sitting, standing, vision, hearing, dexterity and driving requirements.
    - Also include any expected mental demands.

Physical and mental demands:

- Involves sitting approximately 90% of the day, walking or standing the remainder.
- Combination of sitting, standing, bending, light lifting and walking.
- Requires a full range of body motion, including manual and finger dexterity and hand-eye coordination.
- Lifting up to 20 pounds.
- Requires corrected vision and hearing to a normal range.
- Occasional stress from varying demands.

12. **Is this a full time or part time job?**

- Identify the typical work shift, days and overtime expectations

Position type and expected works hours: Full time, business hours, Monday through Friday, but occasional evening, holiday, and weekend work. Some flexibility required. Must be available to have a mixed schedule of opening and closing the office and the ability to be flexible with schedule when needed.

13. **Is travel involved?**

- Candidates need to understand if they are required to travel between clinic locations. Policies will need to be written to outline reimbursement guidelines.
- List percentage of travel time expected, where the travel occurs, and whether it is overnight travel.

Travel: Limited travel, primarily local during business hours. Less than 10% of monthly hours.

14. What is the required education and experience?

- Indicate education based on requirements that are job-related and consistent with business necessity. Remember, job descriptions should not state that a job can only be performed by a licensed or certified professional when that is not actually a requirement of the state.

> **Required Education and Experience:**
>
> - Bachelor's degree.
> - Individuals may also need to complete additional coursework upon hire.
> - Completion of a medical terminology course, or successfully completing one within six months of employment.

15. What is the preferred education and experience?

- Indicate preferred education and experience, but it must relate to this job specifically

> **Preferred Education and Experience:**
>
> - College-level coursework in healthcare administration preferred.
> - Minimum three years of administrative experience, including at least one year of management experience in healthcare

16. What other eligibility qualifications exist?

- List additional licensure or certification necessary to have this job.

> **Additional eligibility qualifications:**
>
> - MGMA or PAHCOM certification.

17. What other duties as assigned?

- There is no way to identify every task in a practice. This is a general disclaimer statement that catches any other assigned duties.

> Please note this job description is not designed to cover or contain a comprehensive listing of activities, duties or responsibilities that are required of the employee for this job. Duties, responsibilities, and activities may change at any time with or without notice.

18. Include two signature lines.

- The employee and hiring manager should sign the job description and date it.

Putting It All Together

Now that you've answered these questions, you have all the components required to create the final job description. A sample job description for an office manager has been created. Keep in mind this is to be used an an illustrative guide only. This job description and all job descriptions provided in this hiring manual will need to be edited to describe the specific requirements your organization has for that role. Include any information that helps make the duties, responsibilities, and expectations for the role clear.

Job title: Office Manager
Classification: Exempt
Reports to Practice Owner Reviewed: 08.01.2019

Summary:
A management position responsible for the daily operations of the medical practice.

Essential Job Responsibilities:

- Enhance patient experiences; optimizing company reputation.
- Ensure compliance with current healthcare regulations, medical laws, federal
  and state laws, and high ethical standards.
- Oversee daily office operations and delegate authority to assigned supervisors.
- Assist supervisors in developing and implementing short- and long-term work plans and objectives for clerical functions.
- Assist supervisors in understanding/implementing clinic policies and procedures.
- Develop guidelines for prioritizing work activities, evaluating effectiveness, and modifying activities as necessary. Ensure that office is staffed appropriately.
- Assist in the recruiting, hiring, orientation, development, and evaluation of clerical staff.
- Establish and maintain an efficient and responsive patient flow system.
- Oversee and approve office supply inventory, ensure that mail is opened and processed, and offices are opened and closed according to procedures.
- Support and uphold established policies, procedures, objectives, quality improvement, safety, environmental and infection control, and codes and requirements of accreditation and regulatory agencies.

Competencies:

Knowledge

- Knowledge of policies and procedures to manage operations and ensure effective patient care.
- Knowledge of the principles and practices of healthcare administration, fiscal management, and government regulations and reimbursements.
- Knowledge of Electronic Health Systems.
- Knowledge of Practice Management Systems.
- Knowledge of medical practices, terminology, and reimbursement policies.
- This position requires strong working knowledge of managed care plans, insurance carriers, referrals, and precertification procedures.

Job title: Office Manager

Skills

- Skill in exercising a high degree of initiative, judgment, and discretion.
- Skill in analyzing situations accurately and taking effective action.
- Skill in establishing and maintaining effective working relationships.
- Skill in organizing work, delegating and achieving goals and objectives.
- Skill in exercising judgment and discretion in developing, interpreting, and implementing departmental policies and procedures.
- Skill in planning and supervising.
- Skill in evaluating the effectiveness of existing methods and procedures.
- Mastery of spoken and written English;

Abilities

- Ability to establish and maintain effective working relationships with other employees and the public.
- Ability to communicate and present information under pressure.
- Ability to read, interpret, and apply clinic policies and procedures.
- Ability to identify problems, recommend solutions, organize and analyze information.
- Ability to establish priorities and coordinate work activities.
- Ability to work independently and be goal-directed.
- Effectively multitask without compromising quality.
- Ability to comprehend and excel in both verbal and written communication, including proper telephone etiquette, face-to-face interactions, and electronic communications.
- Ability to communicate with individuals and small groups with credibility and confidence.

Other

- Willingness and desire to maintain regular and acceptable attendance; may be required to work weekend, holiday, or overtime hours. Must be available to have a mixed schedule of opening and closing the office and the ability to be flexible with schedule when needed.
- Willingness and drive to handle complex, difficult interactions, remain calm under stress, manage emotional situations, display empathy, and maintain positive communication within a rapidly changing/dynamic environment.

Position Type and Expected Works Hours:

Full time, business hours, Monday through Friday, but occasional evening, holiday, and weekend work. Some flexibility required.

Job title: Office Manager

Equipment Operated:

Standard office equipment, including computers, fax machines, copiers, printers, telephones, etc.

Physical and Mental Demands

- Involves sitting approximately 90% of the day, walking or standing the remainder.
- Combination of sitting, standing, bending, light lifting and walking.
- Requires a full range of body motion including manual and finger dexterity and hand-eye coordination.
- Lifting up to 20 pounds.
- Requires corrected vision and hearing to a normal range.
- Occasional stress from varying demands.

Travel:
- No travel is expected for this position.

Required Education and Experience:

- Bachelor's degree,
- Individuals may also need to complete additional coursework upon hire.
- Completion of a medical terminology course or successful completion within six months of employment.

Preferred Education and Experience:

- College-level coursework in healthcare administration preferred.
- At least one year of healthcare administration experience.

Additional Eligibility Qualifications:
- MGMA, PMI, or PAHCOM certification.

Other Duties:

Please note this job description is not designed to cover or contain a comprehensive listing of activities, duties or responsibilities that are required of the employee for this job. Duties, responsibilities and activities may change at any time with or without notice.

Signatures

This job description has been approved by all levels of management:

Manager_____

Employee signature below constitutes employee's understanding of the requirements, essential functions and duties of the position.

Employee_____ Date _____

Wrapping up: Preparing the Job Description

This Office Manager job description is simply a road map. A carefully constructed job description identifies what is negotiable and what isn't for this clinical function. When this important stage of hiring is overlooked, it is much easier to compromise what is needed for the position, which can result in a poor hiring decision. Making poor hiring decisions costs the practice money, creates liability, and results in lost time. Using best practices will mitigate these risks.

It is as important for the candidate to assess the practice as vice versa. A well-written job description can be the perfect communication tool. Although the interview is important for a face to face discussion, it is the job description that is setting the tone for the discussion. It is also one of the best defense tools in employment complaints.

The job description helps ensure that the future employee and the practice are a good fit for each other. It sets the expectations from the beginning and can be used for orientation, feedback sessions, and the annual performance review. A good job description protects both the employer and the employee from unexpected surprises.

So, what's next? It is time to recruit to find the right candidate for the right job.

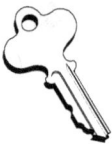

Key Takeaways

- Job descriptions should complement the practice mission.
- Good job descriptions establish the expectations of the candidate, employee, and management.
- It is necessary to know key HR laws when writing job descriptions to protect the practice.

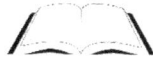

The Recruitment Process Reconsidered

"Hiring the best is your most important task."
Steve Jobs

Recruitment at its core, is a basic, fundamental activity in all businesses. It is a process that if done well will help secure the practice's future. Why is it so important? It's important because it helps solidify the practice's reputation.

Consider this—if you walked into a medical practice for an interview, the front desk was unmanned, they weren't aware you were coming in for an interview, the interview was then conducted haphazardly and unfinished, what would you walk away thinking about that medical practice? Most likely, you would walk away thinking the practice does not know what they are doing, they were disorganized, disorderly, and treated you poorly.

How would you talk about that practice in the future? You, and others, would speak ill of the practice, telling this story possibly years to come. This might just be an interview gone awry and may not be a clear picture of the practice, but the story would linger in a negative way.

How do you rectify this? Using best practices to recruit staff that create the workplace culture you want in your medical practice. If you have recruited properly and filled your open positions with the best fit from a business and culture perspective, your business will thrive.

45

Satisfied employees create a satisfied patient population, which will create a successful practice, according to studies reported by *Forbes*. A successful practice means there is a likelihood that the practice will continue. Business continuity and continuation is vital, without successful caring individuals who think of your business as their business, your practice won't reach its full potential. This impacts not only the sustainability of your practice but the growth and the revenue overall. Your employees are your first line of customer service, excellent customer service will bring your patients and families back time and again.

The Recruitment Process

The recruitment process, from analysis to onboarding, is a costly endeavor. The process takes time and energy to complete in a manner that acquires the best candidates and the best employee. The costs associated with recruitment are extensive, including the time it takes away from your core business, but it is a requirement.[1] In a series of case studies analyzed by the Center for American Progress, it was found that 'quick hiring' could save an employer up to 50% of the employee's annual salary versus a full recruitment drive with analysis—but that there would be a better than 25% chance that within a year employee turnover would cost the company anywhere from 5% up to 213% of the employee's annual salary[2] This is why hiring has to be executed well the first time around. Besides the financial deterrent associated with recruiting and hiring the wrong employee, there are other impacts that will ripple through your entire business in a number of ways—some that cannot be calculated, including:

- decreased productivity,
- turnover,

[1] Bersin, Josh. "Employee Retention Now a Big Issue: Why the Tide has Turned," LinkedIn Influencer, August 16, 2013, https://www.linkedin.com/pulse/20130816200159-131079-employee-retention-now-a-big-issue-why-the-tide-has-turned/
[2] Boushey, Heather and Sarah Jane Glynn. "There Are Significant Business Costs to Replacing Employees," Center for American Progress, November 16, 2012, https://www.americanprogress.org/wp-content/uploads/2012/11/CostofTurnover.pdf

- decreased patients seen,
- delayed service times,
- negative viewpoints from customers and employees,
- not enough resources,
- lower morale,
- gossip, and
- information not shared between staff.

The only way to mitigate these costs is hire right the first time using tried and true methods to bring in the best candidate.

What is your turnover rate?

How many people left your practice last year? (X)

What were the total number of positions last year? (Y)

Divide number who left by the number of positions. (X/Y)

That's your turnover rate—for every role turned over, there is both a replacement cost and a cost to your business for not having that role filled

---

How to start the recruitment process.

After you have completed the analysis and determined your practice's needs, consider both *how* and *where* to recruit.

How will you recruit for this position?

The simplest answer is that recruitment comes from many sources to attract and satisfy diverse candidates. It can also be described as using any way possible that yields the best candidates. Examples of methods include:

- Create a superior hiring package:
  - Offer better compensation than the local market.
  - Offer better benefits (such as health or 401K).
  - Offer better career advancement packages.

- Create a stronger culture fit:
  - Offer a closer knit, more supportive environment.
  - Offer a greater scope of employment-based interests and challenges.
  - Offer ties to the local community.
- Create a better tomorrow:
  - Offer education support.
  - Offer vested interest in the company.
  - Extend expanded benefits (not just health) to include employee families (a matching college fund for kids is a powerful retention tool for top recruits.)
- Create personal satisfaction:
  - Offer challenges tailored to the personality of the recruit.
  - Offer team-based reverse interviews to allow top recruits to "interview" you.
  - Allow for flexibility by allowing the recruit choice in one or more non-key functions (things like local charity drive management or inter-office sports activities).

CAUTION

Using a recruiter or a headhunter is expensive. It can cost in excess of 20% of the annual salary unless you have a retained agreement for the recruiter. Before you hire a recruiter, consider whether or not you can successfully recruit internally.

Where should I recruit from?

There are many places to garner qualified and experienced candidates. The first step is to determine if are you going to recruit for this position yourself without using an agency or a recruiter. If you choose to use a recruiter for this position, confirm the details of the contract. The contract should list and explain the associated costs, such as who has the responsibility to pay for any possible advertising or related out-of-pocket expenses. In addition, the contract should cover

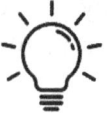

> **Pro Tip:** Ask your current employees for referrals, encourage them to seek out the candidates. Your employees know your workplace, they are well connected, they are your greatest recruiters. For tough to fill roles, incentivize employees with referral bonuses or raffles. Encourage them to post on their social media accounts.

what happens if a candidate applies for the position on their own and is also presented by the recruiter and how to manage previous candidates you've interviewed. It should also address how long the contract period is in place and identify the specific positions for recruitment. Then negotiate who completes the background or licensure verification and references and who your practice works with during the process. These items should be clearly delineated in the contract so you are not haggling or reviewing this after you've found your ideal candidate.

Finding the right candidate on your own is not only possible, but achievable, if you put in the effort. Start by thinking where you want to post the job opening.

The greatest asset you have is your current employee base. Begin by telling your employees the practice has a job opening, then give them a flyer or show them the job posting. Ask your staff for help to fill this job. Be clear with your employees what it is you're looking for in a potential candidate. The more direct you are with your staff, the better the referral will be in the long run. If you need someone who has a specialized degree, tell them. There is nothing worse than having someone referring be told after the fact you were looking for something specific. Don't let your employees put themselves out there with their colleagues or friends only to be embarrassed.

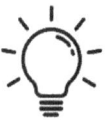

> **Pro Tip:** Look at postings by searching the job title and seeing what others post. This will help you create the best post using keywords and common themes.

Posting an open position is relatively easy now with many little-to-no-cost options. As in all searches, the practice should have a plan to attract the most qualified candidates. Consider postings based on the position, as follows:

- **Create a job posting flyer.** List the who, what, where, when, how, and why of interesting tidbits the candidate will be searching for in their category. Make it appealing, eye catching, and easy to read.
- **Post to job boards like Indeed or ZipRecruiter.** Job boards have low cost models to help small businesses. Indeed also searches for web posts and will link to your job some of the time. Do not count on this, as it does not always happen.
- **Post to LinkedIn.** If your business does not have a LinkedIn account, consider this the ultimate time to start one. Moreover, create one for your practice administrator specifically to post these positions.

Where do you post for the job opening?

- Executive search firms will contact you—make adecision if you wish to do this, if not then proceed with normal recruitment activities .
- Networking—business contacts, community organizations (Rotary Club, Executive Coaches), former business associates.
- Indeed, ZipRecruiter, LinkedIn, Craig's List, local community colleges, local universities/colleges,
- Never underestimate the power of social media and personal relationships for these positions

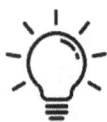

Pro Tip: When posting for the job, if you want to an easy pre-screen, provide the requirements, such as a certification from HFMA or a CPA.

- **Social media.** Is the practice on social media? If so, use the flyer to post this position with a hyperlink for an email or application process.
- **Local schools.** Local universities and/or colleges are an excellent place to connect with job prospects. Alert the career center and/or professors/teachers in this field that you are hiring.
- **Your website.** This is a great place to sell your own organization. Your patients may have referrals and that will speak volumes about your practice!
- **Networking, local organizations, and affiliations.** Are you a member of local organizations or networking group? Do you attend monthly meetings in your field? These are logical places to post these positions and discuss the opening.

You have candidates, now who do you interview?

Most importantly, you must assess the candidates fairly.

- What should you be looking for?
  - Credentials
    - Be fair and equal—it is important to review all candidates equally to avoid any future concerns.
    - Minimum standards—candidates that do not meet the minimum standards will not be prioritied for interviews.
    - Preferred requirements—if applicants meet the preferred requirements, they will be placed at the top of the list for interviews.
    - Skills required for the position—if an applicant meets all the requested skills, the candidate will go to the top for interviews.
  - Job history
    - Assure the job history reflects the skills need for the posted position. It is important to inquire about gaps in the history.

o Instructions

    ❑ Did the applicant follow instructions properly on how to apply? For example, if you requested a salary history and he/she did not provide one, will you exclude the applicant? Perhaps not, but it is good to know your boundaries and what you're willing to waive. This is very important, because if you waive any for one applicant, you must waive it for all.

o Résumé

    ❑ Was the résumé tailored for your position? If it is a generic résumé, does it meet your needs?

o Initiative

    ❑ Did the applicant take initiative by reaching out to the hiring manager or practice administrator?

o Cover letter

    ❑ Did they send one? Is it specific to the job you are posting?

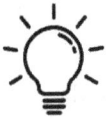

Pro Tip: Create a form to add on top of each résumé to assess each candidate fairly.

Include the following information:

- Candidate Name
- Position Applied For
- Date
- Minimum requirements listed
- Minimum requirements met
- LVN licensed
- CPR certified
- Bilingual
- Interview date

- o Results-oriented
    - ❑ Are the résumé results oriented to showcase their achievements or is it simply a history? This showcases the applicant's work ethic and interest in success.
- o Growth
    - ❑ Is there a history of being moved up, quick growth, or long history of growth? Is the candidate using your practice for growth or to find a home?
- o Competitor
    - ❑ Do they work for a competitor? If so, perhaps you want to interview to get a clearer understanding of the competitor's landscape.

The Application Process

You have now narrowed down your top candidates to interview. The final step in the recruitment process is having an application process that will help you and the candidate carefully discern if offering the position and having it accepted is the right choice for everyone. To best do that, you need to make sure you have an application process that gathers all the pertinent information required.

Do you need an application and a résumé for each applicant?

Absolutely, yes. The résumé is different from an application. The application is a legal document that includes a variety of items that showcase a chronological history of work history, education and skills. Before you interview the candidate, you must have information on each applicant for legal purposes. A résumé is something you will want to have, but it is imperative to have the candidate complete an application.

This is a two-part step that helps the practice get information standardized. All résumés are different and unique to help a candidate stand out to the employer. The application is an equalizer, so all candidates will be judged equally. It gives information about the applicant's background that is not on the résumé. Moreover, the application requires a signature at the end, acknowledging various legal aspects of the interview process. The process allows for more protection for the practice as well.

How do you create an application?

If the practice has a computer-based applicant tracking program, there is a good chance there is an online application process associated with it. Check your system and provider to determine if this is an option. If it is not, there are many samples on the internet to create your own application. The key components[3] to include are as follows:

- Practice name, address, and phone number or use company letterhead
- Applicant's legal name, address, phone number, and email
- Are you eligible to work in the United States? Yes | No
- Are you at least 18 years or older? (If no, you may be required to provide authorization to work.) Yes | No
- Have you ever been terminated from employment or asked to resign by an employer? Yes | No
  - *If yes,* please provide company names and details
- Work History (chronological order with start and end dates) with supervisor name and contact phone number or email along with reason left the employment
- Criminal history
- Salary history
- Educational background
- Preferred schedule (give specific boxes with available day/time combinations)
- How did you hear about us? Walk In | Advertisement | Referral | Other
- Have you ever worked for this company before?
- Do you know anyone who works for our company?
- Reference Listing (3) name, phone number, email, company

[3] Society for Human Resource Management (SHRM) example

- Legal signatures (signing that they understand the practice is an at-will employer)
- It is very important to include something like the following disclosure statement, which the applicant should sign separately:

Please read carefully before signing.

[Practice Name] is an equal opportunity employer. [Practice Name] does not discriminate in employment on account of race, color, religion, national origin, citizenship status, ancestry, age, sex (including sexual harassment), sexual orientation, marital status, physical or mental disability, military status or unfavorable discharge from military service.

I understand that neither the completion of this application nor any other part of my consideration for employment establishes any obligation for [Practice Name] to hire me. If I am hired, I understand that either [Practice Name] or I can terminate my employment at any time and for any reason, with or without cause and without prior notice. I understand that no representative of [Practice Name] has the authority to make any assurance to the contrary.

I attest with my signature below that I have given to [Practice Name] true and complete information on this application. No requested information has been concealed. I authorize [Practice Name] to contact references provided for employment reference checks. If any information I have provided is untrue, or if I have concealed material information, I understand that this will constitute cause for the denial of employment or immediate dismissal.

Date _____ Signature _____

THIS APPLICATION IS VALID ONLY FOR 60 DAYS FROM THE DATE SIGNED/DATED ABOVE.

Wrapping up: Recruitment

Mindful recruitment strategies will be one of the most important commitments you can make to growing the future of your practice culture, teams, and organization. Find ways to introduce consistency into your approach and maximize the potential of your networks and connections. An improved recruitment process can be one of those opportunities where a practice can reap the rewards a seasoned practice manager's persistence and dedication can bring to a problem.

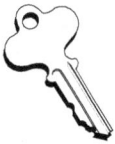

Key Takeaways

- Being consistent in your approach and methodical in your processes will significantly benefit you and your practice or organization in the long run.
- Careful preparation will help you hire the correct candidate.
- A careful application process is the best way to make the seeds of your recruitment efforts bear fruit.

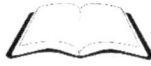

Designing a Hiring Process

"You don't hire for skills, hire for attitude. You can always teach skills." – Simon Sinek

After all the upfront time and energy you took to prepare for the recruitment and application processes, it is time to find the right candidate through a carefully crafted hiring process. This process has a series of fundamental steps, which will be outlined below. By implementing a few best practices, you will be able to refine your process and find the right candidate for your practice.

The Hiring Process

Keep in mind, as you build out your hiring process, that the first and foremost concern is to create a candidate experience that is positive. Aside from any damage the practice's reputation might suffer from word getting around about a poor interview experience, your ideal result is a candidate who very much wants to work for your practice. A carefully crafted process will provide the required structure when the impacts of day-to-day operations might normally cause you to forward in ways that are not ideal.

There will be some steps that will need to be altered depending upon the role being filled. One of those steps is the candidate interview. It can be helpful to have a pre-determined strategy for different types of roles, so that when you have an opening for that type of role, you are clear about your intended interviewing strategy. Similarly, having a pool of questions for those interviews available based on the role will help shorten the time required to prepare for interviews. See Appendix B for some suggested questions based on roles outlined in this hiring manual. Here is a broad outline of the hiring process:

1. Ensure that an applicant tracking system is in place and being followed.

2. Select an interview strategy if one is not already in place.

3. Identify important questions.

4. Prepare the total compensation calculation.

5. Outline ways to understand candidates' alignment with the practice culture.

6. Conduct phone and face-to-face interviews prioritized by candidates who are the best fit for the identified role requirements.

7. Make an offer.

8. Perform pre-employment requirement checks.

9. Communicate with declined applicants.

10. Onboard the new hire.

11. Have a process for reviewing the new hire during the probationary period.

Tracking System for Applicant Information

Most small practices and even larger ones will not have a tracking mechanism or system for tracking the applicants. Some payroll systems have this built in, so make sure to check with your payroll provider. If you don't have an automated system, an Excel spreadsheet is the easiest way track. If you don't have an Excel spreadsheet, you can create something similar in Word or by hand. The spreadsheet/document should include the applicant's name, application date, referred by, interview dates, including any phone interviews. If you have a much larger practice, you may want to invest in an applicant flow tracking system that tracks

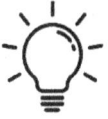

Pro Tip: Retain all applicant information collected and any related hiring notes for a minimum of three (3) years.

Preserve the application information for candidates within a personnel file in a locked filed cabinet behind a locking office door. Personnel file retention regulations vary from state-to-state, so check local/state laws for requirements.

applicants anonymously to help ensure no discrimination has taken place. You will also want to have an organized system for keeping all documents related to the hiring process in a secure location.

No matter how well you think it went, you still might receive a call from the EEOC (Equal Employment Opportunity Commission), the Department of Fair Employment and Housing (DFEH), or directly from a lawyer. This is where having your tracking and documentation in place as you go into the process will help you afterwards. Keep in mind, however, that it is not unusual for the EEOC or DFEH simply to be confirming information they have received. Or they may have an anonymous tip that the practice discriminates against a particular group. This is the moment when you take a *deep breath*, grab your hiring notes, your references, any information you pulled, whatever you did to interview and ultimately fill the position. Anything related from the general period of time when you hired that position should be your focus as you prepare to respond to the complaint.

If you receive a formal complaint, contact an HR consultant or a lawyer before answering the complaint. Time is of the essence. While this may be scary or nerve-wracking, do not delay, as there are specific timeframes for response associated with any complaint.

Considerations for small practices vs large practices

The information needed during a governmental review or if a lawsuit should arise is no different. The size of the organization will only come into play in order to determine if your practice is required to meet additional employment standards. The first magic number is 50; the second is 100. If you have fewer than 50 employees, there is some leeway with the requirements of employment laws. However, you must still treat every applicant with respect and dignity, no matter the size of your practice.

Select the Interviewing Strategy

First, determine the best approach to the interview for the particular role that is being filled. Interview strategies are not a one-size-fits-all decision. Some things to consider to select an interviewing strategy:

Who participates in the interviews?

The default choices tend to be the hiring manager or an HR specialist. Some practices opt to have a couple of interviews with different focuses: an HR specialist narrows down the field, then the hiring manager, then a peer or team member. Another alternative to consider would be a team-based approach. Particularly when roles are tightly embedded in a team-based, collaborative culture, the greatest way to accomplish a successful hire is a group interview. These can offer great insight about the team, the role, and the candidate.

Provide the interviewing team with the job description and meet with them to develop the agenda for the interview and an agreed-upon list of questions. Particularly for staff who have little experience interviewing candidates, thinking through the role, what sort of questions to ask, and who should ask them can help them think more thoroughly about what sort of skills and traits they should be looking for in the interview. It will also give you an opportunity to inform them about appropriate interviewing standards and techniques, and confirm the proposed questions conform to best practices (see the "Formulate the Questions" section of this chapter).

Adding a new team member to any group, can be a stressful and time-consuming. Ensure that the candidate's personality, communication style, and mannerisms will fit with the existing staff. Be cautious that individual nuances are not disguising discrimination but

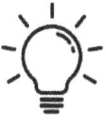

Pro Tip: A phone screening can be a more casual interview; however, there should always be a specific list of questions to structure the interview and provide ease of comparison. Those questions can include:

- Where have you worked?
- Why are you interested in working for our practice?
- What type of job title, work schedule, and salary are you looking for in this role?
- What is prompting the search for a new role?
- When can you start?
- What would you say was your proudest work accomplishment?
- Do you have any questions I can answer?

Phone interviews will usually last from 15 to 30 minutes, depending on the role.

do ensure that the candidate is a complement to the existing staff and is the best fit for your patients. There should be enough similarities that colleagues have things in common, but not so much similarity that the practice loses the benefit of diversity. Team interviews are a great way to experience this fit and discern if the desired synergy is observed.

Use phone interviews to screen applicants

Always complete a phone interview before inviting candidates to your office. An in-person interview takes time, perhaps time that is not available since there is an opening. Conducting a phone interview allows the hiring manager or HR specialist to get a feel for the candidate before committing the time and resourcces to a face-to-face interview. It also allows the for the opportunity to rank applicants to guide the decision on who to invite for the in-person appointments. Phone interviews should be quick confirmations of basic details and a short information-gathering session in order to decide about inviting for an interview. If you've conducted the phone screening and you're not sure if the applicant should come in, let the candidate know you'll be in touch at a later date as you determine the interview schedules.

Take full advantage of the in-person interview

Creating a workplace interview that is positive is similar to creating a practice a patient will want to visit. Below is a possible scenario for setting up the interview for success:

- Invite the applicant to sit down and provide someplace they can wait comfortably. If there is going to be a delay that is any longer than 10 minutes, explain why and thank them for waiting.
- Offer a beverage.
- Provide the candidate with an interview schedule.
- You body language should be relaxed yet energetic. If you are busy and harried, the applicant will feel unwanted or an imposition.
- Treat the candidate respectfully with:
  o Direct eye contact
  o A firm handshake
  o A warm , welcoming smile
- When you invite the applicant into the interview room, make it clear where he or she should sit.
- Give the applicant a tour of the facility, which is an exercise that is useful to you and the applicant, as it is an opportunity to gauge how they fit in the practice environment.)

Formulate the Questions

You will want to prepare a number of questions in advance. Keeping a core list of questions you ask each applicant will ensure uniformity and make later comparisons more equitable. Consider asking behavior-

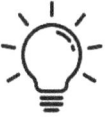

Pro Tip: There are a few simple best practices for face-to-face interview.

- Do *not* write on the applicant's résumé or application; use a pre-filled out paper to attach to the résumé/application.
- Give applicants a tour of the practice. Look for social or normal cues to determine if they have solid customer service skills and will be a good steward for the organization (e.g., o they make eye contact with the employees and with the patients. Do they pick up trash in the hallway? Do they converse while walking them around? Do they stop for conversation with people?)
- In an interview, it is okay for you to be quiet. Allow the applicant to add more to your question and their answer. If their answer is short, encourage them to tell you more.

based questions that can show you the character of candidates: how they will work and integrate into the culture of the practice. The key is to get to an understanding of how a possible candidate will relate to and solve situations with patients and other staff. The best practice for interviewing is to ask open-ended, conversational questions.

A sampling of open-ended questions includes:

- Please tell me about your career and your background.
- What do you know about this practice?
- What makes you the right candidate for this role?
- After walking the practice, what immediately would you want to change?

Some example scenario-based and behavior-based questions

- Tell me about difficulties you experienced in your last position.
- Describe what work environment makes you your most successful.
- What would you change about your last work environment?
- What do you want me to remember about you after this interview?
- Is there anything else I should know about you and your work history or possible work here?

The questions to never, never ask . . . ever

There are many questions that are inappropriate and unlawful to ask while in an interview. Generally, these are questions that pertain to a person's protected class. A protected class is a group of people qualified for special protection by a law, policy, or similar authority. Overall, it is best to avoid questions that are about gender, color, religion, national origin, gender identity, sexual orientation, political affiliation, family status, disability, or the like. These are questions that, if asked, may open up potential for a discriminatory filing or lawsuit.

A sampling of questions that you should **not ask** are listed below. This is **not** a comprehensive list.

DO NOT ASK
Are you married?
Do you plan to have kids?
What does your spouse do?
Where did you grow up?
What year were you born?
Do you have any bankruptcies?
Have you ever filed a worker's compensation claim?
Have you been injured at work before?
Do you normally wear your hair that way?

DO NOT ASK
Do you have a cane you will use when at the office?
How will you manage the wheelchair in the hallway?
If you got the job, how do you get to work?
Who did you vote for?
Are you a Republican or a Democrat?

Things to share about the practice

The interview process is not only a time for the practice to learn about the candidate, it is also a good time to make sure the candidate understands things about practice and organization standards, policies, and procedures. For example, some clinics don't pay mileage if the person travels straight from their home to the alternate clinic but will pay the standard reimbursement rate if change in location occurs during the day. This expectation should be communicated with the candidate during the interviewing stage. Anything that might be an unpleasant surprise on either side including restrictions on paid time off around holidays, dress code standards, or any other concerns the practice has had to manage in the past should be shared. Keeping a list of these items and sharing them with all applicants will protect the practice from the risk of complaints or litigation.

You've Made a Decision

You've done all the hard work and invested considerable effort into finding just the right person for the role and you now have a candidate you would like to bring onto the team. Now what? It is important at this point for the practice to follow the same hiring practices for each new hire, no matter the role. Implementing a few best-practices steps can go a long way in protecting the practice and providing the candidate the fair and equal opportunity they deserve. You may be eager to go ahead and extend an offer and close the deal, but make all final employment decisions contingent upon your all due-diligence verifications, including background checks, OIG clearance, drug screen, education verification, and skills checks.

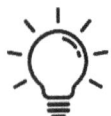

> **Pro Tip:** What to ask during a reference check:
>
> - Verify candidate's employment dates, title, salary (they may not give to you).
> - Ask if the person re-hirable.
> - Ask for their overall impression of the candidate.
> - Inquire if there is anything specific you should know about this candidate.
>
> **CAUTION:** Making a hiring decision based purely on one person's reference-call responses could trigger a complaint if the candidate is not hired.

Reference Checks

It is a good idea to call the candidate's references before making an offer. The candidate should consent to you contacting at least three references. References should consist of former employers, supervisors, or colleagues. Reference questions should be standardized. You should ask each person the same questions and then document the answers in the same way. It is important to confirm dates of employment, job title, duties performed, and reason for separation. Remember that while a former employer can say anything that is factual and accurate, what qualifies as factual and accurate can be difficult to prove. Concern over lawsuits causes many former employers to only confirm position, attached salary, and the dates of employment. Despite this, always ask if there is anything they would like to specifically share with you about the candidate.

> **CAUTION:** Do not disclose specific information the references shared with you if the reference is negative. This is confidential.

Document each call or email for the personnel file. Best practice is to have at least two references checked, previous employment or professional references. In some scenarios, a personal reference may be used, but this would be for an entry-level position or someone with little to no work experience. Whatever information is shared should be between you and the reference provider. It should not be shared with the candidate. Reference check are an excellent first line of defense that may protect your organization from having to endure the pain and costs of a bad hire.

Unfortunately, there are many candidates who are either blatantly dishonest or embellish the truth. It is important to fact check information presented by the candidate. You can use social media as a reference point; however, the practice should have policies around the use of this information. The policies will protect the organization, particularly if the social media research shows that the potential candidate belongs to a protected class. Under no circumstances can a person's class or right to free speech be violated or perceived to be violated in preventing them to be considered for a position. While it may be appealing to check on candidates to confirm they would represent your practice well on social media, unless your policies are explicit, acting upon this information may expose the practice to risks.

> **CAUTION:**
>
> Conducting any type of background check before a formal offer is made to the candidate is not appropriate. Do not ask candidates for any identity-related information (e.g., Social Security, previous names, aliases, etc.) without first making an offer.

Total Compensation

The explanation of compensation can be a difficult conversation, so be prepared before making an offer to paint this complete picture. Particularly if the applicant is in a role with labor pool shortages, it will be that much more important to explain the total compensation for the position. *Total compensation* includes all monies the employee will make in this role, including annualized salary, benefits, vacation time value, 401(k) investments, and educational benefits. This is the opportunity for the practice to show the prospective employee what they will fully earn during their employment on an annual basis.

This matters significantly to an employee, as it is their total picture of what they will earn, in salary as well as benefits. It may be useful for some practices to prepare a "Total Compensation Statement" they can provide to the employee to illustrate the true value of working for the practice. The more detailed information, the more beneficial it will be to the potential employee.

You may want to include the following items in a total compensation statement:

- Annualized pay
  - o If position is hourly, take the hourly rate x 2080 to get this annualized number.
- Medical benefits
  - o Include the amount paid by the employee *and* the employer contribution.
- Flexible spending account
  - o Include details on how this is implemented.
- Paid leave
  - o List all vacation/sick/PTO, holidays, personal days, floating holidays, or whatever else is offered.
- Volunteer opportunities
  - o Describe the volunteer program and recent or near-future projects.
- Disability insurance
  - o Short or long term
- Life insurance
  - o If paid by the practice, show figures.
- Employee Assistance Program
- Educational Assistance or Tuition Reimbursement
  - o Annual amount
- Retirement
  - o 401(k) (include any matching).
- Career pathway or advancement

> **Offer Phone Call Example**
>
> Hello. This is _____ from _____. It was a pleasure meeting you and learning about you. After careful consideration we have decided we'd like to offer you the position of _____. The position would pay $_____ per hour, and we'd like you to start on _____. This offer is contingent upon you meeting a number of pre-employment requirements, including a drug screen, criminal background check, and education verification. If you are still interested in the position, we will send you an offer letter and will need some additional information.

Employment Offers and Offer Letters

Following satisfactory reference checks and a confirmed calculation of total compensation, you've reached the decision to extend an offer of employment. What is next? And how is it conducted? The simplest communication method and a best practice is to call the candidate directly and make a verbal offer.

Written offers of employment—contingent offers

The best practice for any type of employment offer, once a verbal offer is accepted, is to make a formal offer in writing. This is done in order to clarify what is being offered, what the pre-employment requirements are prior to the start date, and what the compensation, benefits, and perks for the position are. The letter should explain the offer is contingent upon satisfactory results returned for your practice's pre-employment requirements. The letter should also cover the hourly salary, paydays, supervisor information, benefit information, the start date(s) of those benefits, and who to contact for more benefits information. It should relay information about orientation, training details, schedule, and any other details that will help the new hire feel ready to go when they walk in the practice door on their first day.

Pre-employment Requirements

Every practice, no matter its size, should have a comprehensive list of pre-employment verifications that are performed before the hire is

71

finalized. The practice will need to clearly communicate with the new hire that their employment offer is contingent on the results of those verifications.

Criminal background checks

Background checks are valubale source of protection for your organization. Although the process will cost money, it is minimal compared to what the unknown can cost. Candidates must consent to their background checks and provide their Social Security number, any previous names or aliases, and the names of counties that are applicable based on the candidate's previous residences. The general rule is to review the past 7 years of criminal history.

A reputable background check company should be able to advise you as to what your state/county/local ordinances allow for background checks. The company you have engaged should be able to guide you and recommend what is a best practice for your organization. If they are unsure or cannot provide what you believe to be credible information, move on to a new company. If you try using an internet search firm without customer service, you will most likely not get the type of background check that will satisfy the due diligence standards you and your practice would require. This type of search will yield simple and basic information that will not pass muster in a state or federal survey.

Pre-employment background checks must be administered in compliance with all federal, state, and local laws and all candidates must be treated equally. Decisions for employment cannot be based on a person's race, national origin, color, sex, religion, disability, genetic information, gender identity, ethnicity, political affiliation, or age. For more specific information, refer to the EEOC website.[1] Keep in mind that a criminal background does not automatically eliminate someone from a job. Make sure that you are not discriminating when considering this information. Sometimes the circumstances may influence your decision of the applicability of this information. If you are unsure about

---

[1] https://www.eeoc.gov/eeoc/publications/background_checks_employers.cfm

a candidate's background, it is best to seek out professional human resources consulting or legal advice.

Regardless of the background check results, treat the candidate with respect by keeping information private and confidential. This information is not intended to be shared with the general office population and should be kept in locked and secured files. This information should only be discarded by shredding the information and should not be disposed of in the regular waste basket. Just as a patient's information is considered private and confidential, the practice should protect any candidate and employee's private information.

HHS OIG clearance

Many background check companies will provide, as part of the standard healthcare background check, the U.S. Department of Health and Human Services Office of Inspector General (HHS OIG)'s listing to confirm the candidate is not on the List of Excluded Individuals/ Entities (LEIE), also known as *the exclusion list*. This is mandatory for clinical personnel and a choice for other personnel, however, best practice says conduct this check for all potential employees. The OIG has the authority to exclude individual from federally funded healthcare programs for a variety of reasons, including a conviction for fraud.[2] This includes any pending investigations being conducted by the OIG. If the background company you contract with does not do this, you must do this prior to day one, but after the contingent offer has been made. Any company or person who hires an individual on the list may be subject to civil monetary penalties. Complete this search yourself by visiting the OIG website as listed below and typing in the candidate's name. Take caution—many people have the same names; it is important to confirm identity when withdrawing a job offer.

Illicit drug screening

Many states require a pre-employment drug screen of all healthcare staff. Make sure to check local and state laws. Again, this is done post-

---

[2] https://oig.hhs.gov/exclusions/index.asp

offer and completed once an employment offer is made. Consent is required to conduct the pre-employment drug screen. Choose a vendor that specializes in pre-employment exams. It is best practice for the candidate to have one attempt for the urine drug screen. In other words, if candidates miss the scheduled appointment, they would automatically be disqualified as an employee of the organization.

Skills checks

If a specific skill has been identified in the job description, it is necessary to validate the information is true. This is precisely why a reference check is important. It gives an opportunity to confirm with a prior employer. If it is a new graduate, the instructor or a clinical site supervisor can be one of the references. If it is a technical skill or language competency, quizzes, assessments, or demonstration may provide the confirmation needed. This will be further reviewed in the section in the chapter on orientation and onboarding of personnel. A new hire will need to demonstrate competency in front of a supervisor or peer. This confirmation should be done prior to a new employee working independently without supervision.

Education, licensure, and certifications verification

All job offers should be made as contingent upon verification of education, licensure, and certification status. In recent years, news stories have reported that prestigious leaders of organizations have falsely claimed to hold degrees required for the positions they were holding. Unfortunately, it happens. To protect the organization, make sure to validate education, training, licensure, and/or certifications via the university, trade school, professional association, or state board conferring the credential. Ultimately, it is the leader's responsibility to ensure that the patients are being seen by qualified individuals.

It is essential to confirm all credentials after the offer, but prior to first day, in order to confirm the applicant's résumé is accurate. While you wouldn't expect a well-respected member of your community to not have an accurate résumé, you would be surprised by the percentage of people who do not put the correct information on their résumé. Confirming credentials differs for each role or position category. Larger organizations may use a service to confirm and validate, but smaller practices will usually complete it by phone or online. Either method works as long as it is completed and documented.

Specifically, for administrative positions, credentials may include:

- Degrees
  - o Doctorate in business or public health
  - o Master's degree in health services administration, business, public administration, health informaiton management, or public health
  - o Bachelor's degree
- Licensure and credentials
  - o CPA for accountants
  - o SHRM for human resources managers
  - o CMPE, CMM, CMOM certifications for practice managers
  - o RHIA, RHIT certifications for health information professionals
- Published information or articles

What if the candidate does not meet the requirements?

Not all candidates will pass the pre-employment requirements. When this happens, it is challenging being the person who must rescind the job offer. The cleanest way to do this is to contact the candidate via phone and explain to them in a concise manner that the pre-employment requirements were not met. Tell them that you're very sorry, but you must rescind the offer, and you wish them the best of luck. Although the candidate will usually have some idea they have issues that might identified during pre-employment screening, it is not unusual for the candidate to nonetheless want specific information. If you utilize a company to complete the background check, you can refer them directly to that company. If you completed the background check yourself, you can share the information you discovered.

Occasionally, the information discovered during a pre-employment screening is false or unsubstantiated, e.g., the OIG has multiple similar names or perhaps the drug screen results are inconclusive. When there are questionable results from any of the pre-employment screening, it is recommended to contact the candidate and explain the situation. This gives candidates an opportunity to explain or rectify any issues identified. This is perfectly acceptable. The key is to provide a timeframe within which candidates must resolve the issues or discrepancies. Your position cannot remain open indefinitely. It is best to give the candidate a two-week period or 10 business days to resolve the issue or the offer is rescinded.

Declining other applicants

Many businesses fail to contact other interviewed candidates. It is a part of the process that no one, even the most skilled professional, wants to do. You are relaying a rejection to the candidate, which is difficult both to offer and receive. It is an uncomfortable but key part to closing out the hiring process. The best course of action is to contact each candidate via phone. The hiring manager or HR representative completing the search should contact the face-to-face candidates once the other candidate has passed all contingencies on their employment.

Onboarding Completes the Hiring Process

Onboarding is the time to bring the new employee into your organization, and it involves new hire orientation, training, and the probationary period. It is the opportunity not only to teach the job but

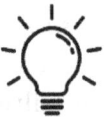

Pro Tip: On an annual basis, all practice employees should be screened against the HHS OIG exclusion list, as this information does change. A suggested process is to run these names, print the results, and place them in a binder or a folder labeled "List of Excluded Individuals Screening for [YEAR]."

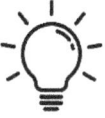

Pro Tip: Calculating the onboarding costs per hire

1. Total pre-employment screening costs per candidate .
2. Number of hours to orient and train multiplied by the hourly rate of the trainer
3. Number of hours to orient and train multiplied by the hourly rate of the new hire.
4. Advertising costs (if any)

Total re-employment screening costs = $85
Trainer time = $25 x 15 hours = $375
New hire time $15 x 15 hours = $225
Advertising costs = $75
—————
Total = $760

This is an incredibly modest and conservative number.

to assimilate the new hire into the practice culture. This is the time to assess their skills hands-on and give them the opportunity to receive the benefit of having supervisor or peer training and guidance. Onboarding is the final piece of the puzzle to having a full-fledged successful member of your team. Proper onboarding is costly; it requires even more effort and time than recruitment. It may be tempting to reduce or eliminate it. But keep in mind that according to the Society for Human Resources Management (SHRM), 69% of employees are more likely to stay with a company for three years if they experienced great onboarding.[3] The majority of employees fail in the first 90-days of employment due to poor onboarding. A survey conducted by Allied Workforce Mobility discovered that companies lose 25% of all new employees within the first year.[4]

---

[3] Maurer, Roy. 2015, April 15. *Onboarding Key to Retaining, Engaging Talent.* Retrieved from https://www.shrm.org/resourcesandtools/hr-topics/talent-acquisition/pages/onboarding-key-retaining-engaging-talent.aspx.

[4] Allied Workforce Mobility Survey. 2012, March. Retrieved from http://hriq.allied.com/pdfs/AlliedWorkforceMobilitySurvey.pdf.

Make sure to have made all the arrangements and generated the necessary materials to properly onboard the new hire, including employee handbooks, training schedules, peer mentors information, before the new hire's first day. No one benefits from a last-minute scramble added to the already challenging practice environment. Take the time to discuss the onboarding process experience with employees once they complete the probationary stage and be prepared to implement improvements based on that feedback.

Probationary Period

A probationary period is the time the practice has determined is the training period required for the new employee to be successful in that role. A probationary period is generally 90-days. However, this does not mean you simply terminate the employee if they aren't doing a good job. That is not the intention of the probationary period. From day one of the probationary period, the practice should invest in training, assessing, and providing active feedback on the work product of the new employee. It is the supervisor's responsibility to accurately train and develop the new employee. The supervisor should supervise this employee by giving them the tools to be successful, answer questions, follow up on the day's work, and check in every day/week/month to assure the new employee understands and is completing their job assignments properly. The new employee should not at any time be wondering how they are doing in their new job; the supervisor must communicate this on at least a weekly basis, if not daily.

Be prepared for the new hire to struggle at points. It can be helpful to assign a peer mentor if possible or find another way to provide support.Not only will the new hire need support, but the staff will also be adjusting to a new teammate during this period.

Wrapping up: Hiring

The hiring process is the last chance for the candidate and the practice to determine mutual fit. Does the candidate fit the role as far as knowledge, skills, abilities, and attitude? Does the candidate fit with the team and practice culture? Is the role going to be the right one for the candidate?

Answering these key questions is pivotal to the success of the hire, the success of the team, and the success of the practice going forward.

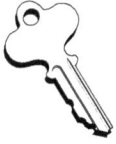

Key Takeaways

- Create a positive candidate experience.
- There are many regulations around the hiring process. Be sure everyone involved has been educated on them, and the practices policies designed to mitigate risk. Don't hesitate to consult an HR specialist.
- Don't waste all the hiring effort by failing to properly train and onboard the new hire. A sink or swim philosophy is not goingn to create success for the new hire or the practice.

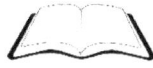

Summary

"Hiring people is a form of investing. You have to do your research and make sure you're spending your resources on the right pick." – Warren Buffett

The most important outcome of careful hiring processes is to have an employee base that shares the vision the leadership has for the practice. These employees will represent the practice for a long time. Keep the following points in mind:

- Treat everyone equally and fairly.
- Do not rush the hiring process.
- Prepare the new employee for success with a careful onboarding process.

Hopefully, hiring is not an everyday occurrence in your medical practice. But when it becomes necessary, this guide is available to help remind about best practices. In addition, it will help the practice be more prepared to place the right resources at the right time. Falling short in the hiring process will only lead to turnover in the position and may well have an effect throughout the entire organization. Healthcare is about delivering quality care to patients. Let's put the right people in the right place for the right reasons.

"Always treat your employees exactly as you want them to treat your best customers." – Stephen Covey

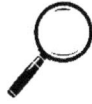

Appendix A
Job Descriptions

Job Title: Phlebotomist

Department: Patient Care

Immediate Supervisor Title: Patient Care Director

Job Supervisory Responsibilities: Nursing and Support Staff

General Summary:

A position responsible for performing venipuncture on patients.

Essential Job Responsibilities:

- Prepares equipment to efficiently collect blood products.
- Performs venipuncture, arterial and capillary punctures on patients as directed by physician and following medical practice protocols related to safety, infection control, and confidentiality. Conducts laboratory tests on specimens.
- Enters data into computer.
- Enhance patient experiences; optimizing company reputation.
- Ensure compliance with current healthcare regulations, medical laws, federal and state laws, and high ethical standards.
- Maintain patient flow.
- Assists patient before, during, and after blood draw.
- Instructs on urine collection procedures.
- Cleans/sterilizes equipment, instruments, and work area following safety, cleanliness, and infection control procedures.
- Inventories supplies and places orders to ensure adequate supplies for procedures.

Education:

- High school diploma or equivalent.

- Graduation from an accredited medical vocational institution with phlebotomy course diploma.
- National certification through American Medical Technologists as a registered phlebotomy technician not required but helpful.
- Current CPR certificate.

Experience:

- 1-2 years medical experience is preferred, but not required.
- Minimum one year of phlebotomy experience.
- Medical practice experience helpful.

Other Requirements:

- Willingness to work with underprivileged populations.
- Must have sympathetic attitude toward the care of the ill.
- Must be available to have a mixed schedule of opening and closing the office and the ability to be flexible with schedule when needed.
- MGMA certification.
- Satisfactory completion of background checking process.
- Willingness to adhere to stated program and documentation protocols.
- ASCP required; certification as medical assistant preferred but not required.

Competency requirements:

Knowledge

- Knowledge of phlebotomy techniques.
- Knowledge of clinic protocols and policies.

Skills:

- Skill in performing efficient and effective draws.

- Skill in conducting cooperative interactions with patients and staff.

Abilities:

- Ability to interpret and respond appropriately to instructions.
- Ability to coordinate eye–hand movements to ensure patient comfort during blood draws.

Equipment Operated:

- Blood draw equipment including syringes, tubes, bandages, and other appropriate supplies.

Work Environment:

Performs duties in medical exam/procedure rooms.
Exposure to communicable diseases, sharp instruments, bodily fluids, cleaning chemicals.

Mental/Physical Requirements:

- Lifting—Not to exceed 50 lbs.
- Writing, Sitting, Bending, Visual acuity, Reading, Field of vision/peripheral
- Standing—spends majority of the shift working on their feet
- Regularly required to use hands to finger, handle, or feel objects, tools, or controls; bend, reach with hands and arms; stoop, kneel, and talk and/or hear.
- Exposure to: Noise, Chemical vapors, Infectious Materials
- Combination of sitting, standing, bending, light lifting and walking.
- Requires a full range of body motion including manual and finger dexterity and hand-eye coordination.
- Requires corrected vision and hearing to a normal range.
- Requires the ability to manage stressful situations.

- Occasional stress from medical situations.

Disclaimer: This description is intended to provide only basic guidelines for meeting job requirements. Responsibilities, knowledge, skills, abilities, and working conditions may change as needs of the organization evolve and on an organization by organization basis.

Job Title:: Laboratory Technician
Department: Laboratory
Immediate Supervisor Title: Laboratory Manager
Job Supervisory Responsibilities:

General Summary:

The **Laboratory Technician** functions as an interdisciplinary team member that performs a wide range of services in clinic and hospital based laboratories such as specimen collection, specimen processing, reception desk duties, scheduling/billing functions, waived point of care laboratory testing, assisting with difficult INT sticks, and a variety of other services unique to the individual work area.

The **Laboratory Technician** is responsible for specimen receipt, identification verification, processing, shipping and storage. Process large volumes of specimens for multiple laboratory testing sites and accurately prepares lab specimens and containers with reagents as required for the ordered testing.

Must be able to prioritize the workload in response to the specific needs of numerous requests. Works with various computer information systems on a daily basis.

Must use critical thinking skills and participate in quality control programs within the laboratory.

Ensures that all services are carried out according to established directions and guidelines in the Procedure Manual designated by The Clinic Laboratory Department.

Interacts with the patient, family, physicians, allied health staff, and visitors as a professional member of the laboratory team.

Essential Job Responsibilities:

- Ensure compliance with current healthcare regulations, medical laws, federal and state laws, and high ethical standards.

Education:

- High school diploma or GED required.
- Associates degree and coursework in a healthcare or science related field is preferred

Experience:

Other Requirements:

- Certification in phlebotomy and one year experience in a clinical laboratory environment with experience at venous access and specimen processing preferred or certification as a Medical Assistant.

Competency requirements:

Knowledge

- Knowledge of laboratory functions, medical terminology, a background in science and 1-2 years medical experience is preferred, but not required.
- Previous experience or knowledge of computers and keyboarding, telephone operations and other office equipment desired.
- Ability to accurately read specimen labels and work with numbers
- to prevent mislabeling.
- Must be organized, able to prioritize and work in a fast-paced
- environment.
- Must possess good human relations skills and be able to communicate effectively both orally and in written form.

- Must be able to work independently as well as in a team environment.
- Must be able to accommodate scheduling adjustments, off-shifts, holiday, and weekend work assignments.
- Requires the ability to be attentive to details and to adhere to strict safety requirements for handling infectious agents.

Skills:

- Must be adaptable and well organized.
- Able to work independently as well as with a team.
- Must have good interpersonal skills when working with physicians, co-workers, and patients. Must be able to accurately read specimen labels and follow standard operating procedures. In addition, must be capable of doing general troubleshooting and problem solving regarding laboratory procedures.
- Works flexible hours to meet workload demands and accommodates schedule changes.
- Must have meticulous attention to detail.
- Ability to communicate in English, both verbally and in writing.
- Additional languages preferred.

Abilities:

- Must maintain regular and acceptable attendance; may be required to work weekend, holiday or OT hours.
- Ability to establish and maintain effective working relationships with other employees.
- Ability to work under pressure, communicate and present information.
- Ability to read, interpret, and apply clinic policies and procedures.
- Ability to identify problems, recommend solutions, organize and analyze information.
- Ability to establish priorities and coordinate work activities.

- Ability to work independently, be goal-directed and have strong organizational skills.
- Effectively multitask without compromising quality.
- Ability to communicate with individuals and small groups with credibility and confidence.
- Ability to handle difficult situations, remain calm under stress, manage emotional situations, display empathy and maintain positive communication during a rapidly changing/dynamic environment.
- Turn problems into opportunities by developing innovative and creative solutions.
- Demonstrate a friendly, positive attitude, display energy and drive in performing daily responsibilities.
- Must be flexible as well as easily adapt to a changing work environment which will require ongoing maintenance of job-related skills/activities.

Equipment Operated:

- Various and diverse laboratory equipment and machinery.

Work Environment:

Position is in a well-lighted laboratory environment. Occasional evening and weekend work.

Mental/Physical Requirements:

- Lifting—Not to exceed 50 lbs.—local practice may apply.
- Writing , Sitting, Standing—spends majority of the shift working on their feet
- Bending Visual acuity, Reading
- Field of vision/peripheral
- Regularly required to use hands to finger, handle, or feel objects, tools, or controls; bend, reach with hands and arms; stoop, kneel, and talk and/or hear.

- Exposed to: Noise, Chemical vapors, Infectious Materials.
- Requires the ability to manage stressful situations.
- Occasional stress from varying demands.

Disclaimer: This description is intended to provide only basic guidelines for meeting job requirements. Responsibilities, knowledge, skills, abilities, and working conditions may change as needs of the organization evolve and on an organization by organization basis.

Job Title: Director of Nursing
Department: Nursing
Immediate Supervisor Title: CEO
Job Supervisory Responsibilities: All the Nurses

General Summary:

An executive position responsible for all nursing staff and clinical nursing operations. May also have administrative responsibility for risk management, utilization management, reimbursement, and specific specialties such as critical care, cardiac care, women's health, or surgical units depending on the services offered by the medical practice.

Essential Job Responsibilities:

- Participates at senior-management level in all planning, budgeting, policy making, and decision making related to clinical operations involving nursing staff.
- Ensures that nursing aspects related to risk management, reimbursement, financial management, and other administrative functions are incorporated into operational systems.
- Monitors outcomes, budget results, patient satisfaction surveys, and other indicators of nursing performance.
- Establishes a human resources plan for nursing including need for numbers and types of nurses and related allied health staff.
- Works with human resources specialist and nurse managers and team leaders to recruit, select, orient, and train new staff.
- Makes sure the performance and productivity of all nursing staff are evaluated on a regular basis throughout the year and annually.
- Advises on appropriate corrective actions and development opportunities.

- Maintains high quality of care by nursing staff through continuous improvement of standards and protocols.
- Ensures all staff are trained in quality assurance/control requirements and meet these standards.
- Stays current with state, federal, and payer regulations/requirements and updates professional standards for nursing for the medical practice appropriately.

Education:

- BSN required; MSN preferred or master's in business, health administration or other related field.

Experience:

- Minimum 10 years of nursing experience with progressively increasing management/operations experience.

Other Requirements:

- Must have sympathetic attitude toward the care of the ill.
- The ANA Nursing: Scope and Standards of Practice provide a basis for the practice of the RN.
- Must be available to have a mixed schedule of opening and closing the office and the ability to be flexible with schedule when needed.
- MGMA certification.
- Current state RN license.
- Current CPR certification.

Competency requirements:

Knowledge

- Knowledge of laboratory functions, medical terminology, a background in science and 1-2 years medical experience is preferred, but not required.

- Previous experience or knowledge of computers and keyboarding, telephone operations and other office equipment desired.
- Ability to accurately read specimen labels and work with numbers to prevent mislabeling.
- Must be organized, able to prioritize and work in a fast-paced environment.
- Must possess good human relations skills and be able to communicate effectively both orally and in written form.
- Must be able to work independently as well as in a team environment.
- Must be able to accommodate scheduling adjustments, off-shifts, holiday, and weekend work assignments.
- Requires the ability to be attentive to details and to adhere to strict safety requirements for handling infectious agents.

Skills:

- Ability to communicate in English, both verbally and in writing.
- Additional languages preferred.
- Must be able to work independently and in a team environment.
- Addressing and rectifying patient and/or staff concerns.
- High-level problem solving skills with flexible solutions for a changing healthcare market.
- Uses VMPS to identify a problem, route cause, and engages the team in solutions.
- Able to navigate through multiple electronic applications and devices, medical equipment, examples include iPad/tablets, Text Reminder notifications.

Abilities:

- Must maintain regular and acceptable attendance; may be required to work weekend, holiday or OT hours.
- Ability to read, write and carry out directions.

- Ability to assemble, maintain and record data in an accurate record.
- Must strictly adhere to safety protocols to work with infectious specimens, chemicals and other hazards.
- Must be capable of producing accurate results under time constraints, multi-tasking, and performing in a fast-paced and changing environment.
- Ability to establish and maintain effective working relationships with other employees.
- Ability to work under pressure, communicate and present information.
- Ability to read, interpret, and apply clinic policies and procedures.
- Ability to identify problems, recommend solutions, organize and analyze information.
- Ability to establish priorities and coordinate work activities.
- Ability to work independently, be goal-directed and have strong organizational skills.
- Effectively multitask without compromising quality.
- Ability to communicate with individuals and small groups with credibility and confidence.
- Ability to handle difficult situations, remain calm under stress, manage emotional situations, display empathy and maintain positive communication during a rapidly changing/dynamic environment.
- Turn problems into opportunities by developing innovative and creative solutions.
- Demonstrate a friendly, positive attitude, display energy and drive in performing daily responsibilities.
- Must be flexible as well as easily adapt to a changing work environment which will require ongoing maintenance of job-related skills/activities.

Equipment Operated:

- Various and diverse healthcare equipment and machinery.
- Networked computer

Work Environment:

Position is in a well-lighted clinical environment.
Occasional evening and weekend work.

Mental/Physical Requirements:

- Lifting—Not to exceed 50 lbs.
- Writing, Sitting, Bending, Visual acuity, Reading, Field of vision/peripheral
- Standing—spends majority of the shift working on their feet
- Regularly required to use hands to finger, handle, or feel objects, tools, or controls; bend, reach with hands and arms; stoop, kneel, and talk and/or hear.
- Exposure to: Noise, Chemical vapors, Infectious Materials
- Combination of sitting, standing, bending, light lifting and walking.
- Requires a full range of body motion including manual and finger dexterity and hand-eye coordination.
- Requires corrected vision and hearing to a normal range.
- Requires the ability to manage stressful situations.
- Occasional stress from medical situations.

Disclaimer: This description is intended to provide only basic guidelines for meeting job requirements. Responsibilities, knowledge, skills, abilities, and working conditions may change as needs of the organization evolve and on an organization by organization basis.

Job Title: Sonographer/Ultrasonographer
Department: Laboratory
Immediate Supervisor Title: Laboratory Manager
Job Supervisory Responsibilities:

General Summary:

A position responsible for using diagnostic medical equipment to diagnose various medical conditions.

May specialize in obstetric/gynecologic, abdominal, neurosonography, or breast sonography.

Essential Job Responsibilities:

- Reviews patient's medical history and physician's instructions.
- Prepares equipment for procedure.
- Selects appropriate equipment settings.
- Enhance patient experiences; optimizing company reputation.
- Ensure compliance with current healthcare regulations, medical laws, federal and state laws, and high ethical standards.
- Maintain patient flow.
- Explains procedure to patient and records any medical history that may be relevant to the condition being viewed.
- Directs the patient to move into positions that will provide the best view.
- Spreads gel on the skin to aid the transmission of sound waves.
- Operates special equipment to direct nonionizing, high-frequency sound waves into areas of the patient's body.
- The equipment collects reflected echoes and forms an image that may be videotaped, transmitted, or

photographed for interpretation and diagnosis by a physician.

- Views the screen during the scan, looking for visual cues that contrast healthy areas with unhealthy ones.
- Selects images to show to the physician for diagnostic purposes.
- Takes measurements, calculates values, and analyzes the results in preliminary reports for the physicians.
- Keeps patient records and adjusts/maintains equipment.
- Complies with safety, infection control, and quality improvement policies/ procedures.

Education:

- Associate's or bachelor's degree in sonography from accredited school.
- Training may be available in hospitals, vocational-technical institutions, and the Armed Forces.

Experience:

- Minimum one or more years of experience and/or training with graduate sonographer.

Other Requirements:

Must be available to have a mixed schedule of opening and closing the office and the ability to be flexible with schedule when needed.

MGMA certification.

No state license required; Certification of competency and registration available through organizations such as the American Registry for Diagnostic Medical Sonography. Registration requires passing a general physical principles and instrumentation examination, in addition to passing an exam in a specialty such as ob/gyn sonography, abdominal sonography, or neurosonography.

Competency Requirements:

Knowledge:

- Knowledge of anatomy, physiology, instrumentation, basic physics, patient care, and medical ethics.
- Knowledge of mathematics and science.
- Knowledge of safety, infection control, and quality improvement practices.

Skills:

- Skill in communication and interpersonal interactions.
- Skill in performing mathematical and scientific calculations.
- Skill in gathering and analyzing patient data.

Abilities:

- Ability to explain technical procedures and results to patients in user-friendly **manner.**
- Ability to calm patients who may be nervous about the procedure.
- Ability to use correct body mechanics to assist patients appropriately.

Equipment Operated:

- Standard office equipment including computers, fax machines, copiers, printers, telephones, etc.
- Variety of sonography equipment including ultrasound machines, transducers, gels, and computer hardware/software.

Work Environment:

- Position is in a well-lighted clinical environment.
- Occasional evening and weekend work.
- Combination of exam and laboratory rooms and darkroom.
- In some situations, may work in operating room.

- Sometimes works in close quarters.
- Exposure to communicable diseases, biohazards, and other conditions related to clinic settings.

Mental/Physical Requirements:

- May be standing for long periods and may have to lift/ turn disabled patients.
- Work primarily at diagnostic imaging machines involving standing, sitting, walking, bending, lifting, and reaching.
- Some stress related to dealing with anxious patients.

Disclaimer: This description is intended to provide only basic guidelines for meeting job requirements. Responsibilities, knowledge, skills, abilities, and working conditions may change as needs of the organization evolve and on an organization by organization basis.

Job Title: X-Ray Technician

Department: Laboratory

Immediate Supervisor Title: Laboratory Manager

Job Supervisory Responsibilities:

General Summary:

A position responsible for operating X-ray and fluoroscopic equipment that assists radiologists and/or physicians with diagnosing and/or treating disease and/or injury.

Essential Job Responsibilities:

- Prepares patients for radiologic procedures.
- Protects patient, self, and other staff from radiation hazards.
- Takes X-rays following established procedures for patient care and safety, which involves setting up and operating radiographic equipment used in the medical diagnosis and/or treatment of patients and includes implementing infection control procedures for the work area.
- Enhance patient experiences; optimizing company reputation.
- Ensure compliance with current healthcare regulations, medical laws, federal and state laws, and high ethical standards.
- Maintain patient flow.
- Selects proper ionizing factors for radiological diagnosis.
- Adjusts/sets radiographic controls.
- Positions patients and takes X-rays of specific parts of the patient's body as requested by physicians.
- Processes film.
- Checks X-rays for clarity of image, retaking when needed.
- Distributes X-rays to appropriate medical staff.

- Maintains required records including patient records, daily log books, and monthly reports. Performs quantity and quality control checks to assure X-ray unit meets standards required by laws, rules, and departmental policies.
- Complies with safety standards.
- Cleans, maintains, and makes minor adjustments to radiographic equipment, including determining equipment repairs.
- Maintains radiographic supplies, film, and orders as necessary.

Education:

- Associate's degree in radiological technology from accredited X-ray technician program.

Experience:

- One to three years of experience as X-ray technician, preferably in medical practice environment.

Other Requirements:

- American Registry of Radiologic Technologists registration preferred.
- Must be available to have a mixed schedule of opening and closing the office and the ability to be flexible with schedule when needed.
- MGMA certification.

Competency Requirements:

Knowledge:

- Knowledge of X-ray procedures and protocols.
- Knowledge of anatomy and physiology necessary to perform X-ray testing including body mechanics and patient movement.

- Knowledge of radiology equipment including safety hazards common to radiology.

Skills:

- Skill in positioning patients properly.
- Skill in identifying equipment problems and correcting or notifying supervisor.
- Skill in following infection control and radiological safety procedures.

Abilities:

- Ability to lift and position patients for the type of X-ray procedure required.
- Ability to notice detail in drawings and differences in shapes and shadings.
- Ability to apply written instructions and standardized work practices.

Equipment Operated:

- Standard office equipment including computers, fax machines, copiers, printers, telephones, etc.
- Radiological equipment used for medical diagnosis and treatment.

Work Environment:

Position is in a well-lighted Clinic environment.
Occasional evening and weekend work.
Radiological unit. Exposure to disease, radiation, and toxic chemicals in the course of performing the work.

Mental/Physical Requirements:

- Standing six to eight hours per day, walking, stooping, and bending.
- Requires ability to move equipment and transfer patients.
- Occasional stress when working with anxious patients.

Disclaimer: This description is intended to provide only basic guidelines for meeting job requirements. Responsibilities, knowledge, skills, abilities, and working conditions may change as needs of the organization evolve and on an organization by organization basis.

Job Title: Respiratory Therapist

Department: Clinical Services

Immediate Supervisor Title: Nursing Supervisor, Attending Physician

Job Supervisory Responsibilities: None

General Summary:

A clinical position responsible for evaluating, treating, and caring for patients with breathing or other cardiopulmonary disorders under the direction of a physician.

Therapists have more responsibility than technicians.

Essential Job Responsibilities:

- Evaluates and treats all types of patients, ranging from premature infants whose lungs are not fully developed to elderly people whose lungs are diseased.
- Interviews patients and performs limited physical examinations.
- Conducts diagnostic tests including checking breathing capacity and determining the concentration of oxygen and other gases in patients' blood.
- Measures patients' pH, which indicates the acidity or alkalinity of the blood.
- Treats patients using oxygen or oxygen mixtures, chest physiotherapy, and aerosol medications. May use oxygen mask or nasal cannula on the patient and set the oxygen flow at the level prescribed by the physician.
- Enhance patient experiences; optimizing company reputation.
- Ensure compliance with current healthcare regulations, medical laws, federal and state laws, and high ethical standards.
- Maintain patient flow.

- Perform various patient care activities and related nonprofessional services necessary in personal needs and comforts of patients.
- Set an example for and reinforcing evidence-based practices.
- Performs chest physiotherapy on patients to remove mucus from their lungs and make it easier for them to breathe.
- Administers aerosols, which are liquid medications suspended in a gas that forms a mist that is inhaled.
- Teaches patients how to inhale the aerosol properly to ensure its effectiveness.
- Teaches patients and their families to use ventilators and other life-support systems at home. May visit patients at home to inspect and clean equipment and to ensure its proper use.
- Complies with safety, infection control, and quality improvement policies and practices. Documents patient care for medical records.

Education:

- Associate's degree in respiratory therapy or cardiopulmonary technology from an accredited school required. Higher level degrees are preferred.

Experience:

- Minimum one year of respiratory therapy experience in acute care setting required.
- Minimum six months of experience in diagnostic testing required.
- Minimum six months of medical practice experience preferred.

Other Requirements:

- Must have sympathetic attitude toward the care of the ill.

- Must be available to have a mixed schedule of opening and closing the office and the ability to be flexible with schedule when needed.
- MGMA certification.
- Most states require respiratory therapists to obtain a license.
- Passing the certified respiratory therapist exam qualifies respiratory therapists for state licenses.

Competency Requirements:

Knowledge:

- Knowledge of human anatomy, physiology, pathophysiology, chemistry, physics, microbiology, pharmacology, and mathematics.
- Knowledge of therapeutic and diagnostic procedures and tests, equipment, patient assessment, and cardiopulmonary resuscitation.
- Knowledge of techniques for teaching patients how to care for themselves outside of clinic.

Skills:

- Skill in applying clinical practice guidelines, cardiac and pulmonary rehabilitation, respiratory health promotion, and disease prevention.
- Skill in medical record keeping to measure patient progress.
- Skill in safe use of respiratory therapy equipment including adherence to safety precautions and regular maintenance and testing of equipment to minimize the risk of injury

Abilities:

- Ability to teach patients and families about using respiratory therapy equipment and techniques at home and in other nonclinical locales.

- Ability to collaborate effectively with physicians and other clinicians.
- Ability to deal compassionately with anxious patients who may have life-threatening illnesses.

Equipment Operated:

- Variety of respiratory therapy equipment including oxygen equipment, ventilators, pulmonary measurement instruments, blood draw equipment, and suction equipment.

Work Environment:

Various laboratory, exam, and office settings.
Trained to work with hazardous gases stored under pressure.
Exposure to communicable diseases, biohazards, and other conditions related to clinical environment.

Mental/Physical Requirements:

- Long hours involving standing, bending, and walking.
- May have to deal with stressful emergency situations.
- Occasional need to lift/carry up to 50 pounds.
- Some stress related to dealing with anxious patients.

Disclaimer: This description is intended to provide only basic guidelines for meeting job requirements. Responsibilities, knowledge, skills, abilities, and working conditions may change as needs of the organization evolve and on an organization by organization basis.

> **Job Title: Social Worker**
>
> **Department: Patient Care**
> **Immediate Supervisor Title: Patient Care Director**
> **Job Supervisory Responsibilities: Nursing and Support Staff**

General Summary:

A nonclincal position responsible for providing professional social work services to patients and families including direct counseling services, crisis intervention, and coordination of community services/resources.

Performance of duties may be autonomous and self-directed as part of an interdisciplinary team.

Essential Job Responsibilities:

- Conducts comprehensive, culturally sensitive psychosocial assessments, develops care plans, and provides counseling and crisis intervention services to individuals and families.
- Enhance patient experiences; optimizing company reputation.
- Ensure compliance with current healthcare regulations, medical laws, federal and state laws, and high ethical standards.
- Coordinates services with appropriate clinic and community resources.
- Provides information and education about health/ mental health issues to individual patients and to groups.
- Documents assessment, intervention, and treatment data in medical record.
- Provides social work consultation to clinic staff and community providers as appropriate.
- Serves as liaison to community health care network.

Education:

- Master's degree in social work from accredited school of social work.
- Additional course work in area of specialty preferred.

Experience:

- Minimum two years of experience in social work and broad background with diverse patient populations, preferably in medical setting.
- Additional one year of experience in area of specialty preferred.

Other Requirements:

- Willingness to work with underprivileged populations.
- Must have sympathetic attitude toward the care of the ill.
- Must be available to have a mixed schedule of opening and closing the office and the ability to be flexible with schedule when needed.
- MGMA certification.
- Satisfactory completion of background checking process.
- Willingness to adhere to stated program and documentation protocols.
- Registered to practice social work in state and/or a current state social work license.

Competency Requirements:

Knowledge:

- Knowledge of professional social work principles, methodology, and ethics and of human psychosocial development within the family, community, and culture.
- Knowledge of the use of therapeutic relationship to foster patient involvement. Familiarity with brief therapy theories/techniques and therapeutic process.

Understanding of techniques for facilitating client motivation to change behavior.

- Knowledge of health and social issues impacting diverse clients and their well-being.

Skills:

- Skill in crisis intervention.
- Skill in client advocacy.
- Skill in case management.

Abilities:

- Ability to interact effectively as member of interdisciplinary health care team.
- Ability to identify and utilize community resources.
- Ability to communicate appropriately with diverse patient population.

Equipment Operated:

- Standard office equipment including computer hardware and software to access community resource database.

Work Environment:

Office and exam room settings. Some exposure to communicable diseases. Some interactions in community provider network/settings.

Mental/Physical Requirements:

- Combination of sitting, standing, and walking.
- Occasional stress in balancing multiple demands and in dealing with patients/families experiencing tension.

Disclaimer: This description is intended to provide only basic guidelines for meeting job requirements. Responsibilities, knowledge, skills, abilities, and working conditions may change as needs of the organization evolve and on an organization by organization basis.

> **Job Title: Medical Assistant**
>
> **Department: Clinical**
>
> **Immediate Supervisor Title: Clinical Manager**
>
> **Job Supervisory Responsibilities: Support staff**

General Summary:

Medical assistants are a crucial component to your practice's clinical staff, but their roles can vary in breadth depending on the size of your practice and the amount of work your physicians, physician assistants and nurses choose to give them.

Essential Job Responsibilities:

- Report to clinical coordinator or practice administrator
- Perform nursing procedures under supervision of physician or physician assistant
- Assist physician and physician assistant in exam rooms
- Escort patients to exam rooms, interviews patients, measure vital signs, including weight, blood pressure, pulse, temperature, and document all information in patient's chart
- Give instructions to patients as instructed by physician or physician assistant
- Ensure all related reports, labs and information is filed is available in patients' medical records prior to their appointment
- Keep exam rooms stocked with adequate medical supplies, maintain instruments, prepare sterilization as required
- Take telephone messages and provide feedback and answers to patient/physician/pharmacy calls
- Triage and process messages from patients and front office staff to physicians and physician assistants

- Maintain all logs and required checks (i.e. refrigerator temperatures, emergency medications, expired medications, oxygen, cold sterilization fluid change, etc.)
- All other duties as assigned by clinical coordinator or practice administrator
- Keep in mind that the responsibilities of your medical assistants will also vary based on practice location, as the legal scope of practice varies by state. For example, some states require medical assistants who perform certain procedures, such as blood draws, ultrasounds or EKGs, to have license to do so, while some states do not. Many practices leave it up to the physician to make decisions about a medical assistant's scope of responsibility, since they are technically working under the license of the physician.

Education:

- High school diploma; some college preferred
- Medical assistant certification (if applicable)
- Maintains BLS (Basic Life Support) for Health Care Providers from one of the following programs:
  - American Heart Association
  - American Red Cross

Other Requirements:

- Must have sympathetic attitude toward the care of the ill.
- Must be available to have a mixed schedule of opening and closing the office and the ability to be flexible with schedule when needed.
- MGMA certification.

Competency requirements:

Knowledge:

- Healthcare field and medical specialty.
- Medical terminology.
- Grammar, spelling, and punctuation.
- Knowledge of EHRs (if applicable).

Skills:

- Exceptional customer service and phone etiquette.
- Ability to maintain effective and organized systems to ensure timely patient flow.
- The ability to perform phlebotomy and administer injections.

Abilities:

- Must maintain regular and acceptable attendance; may be required to work weekend, holiday or OT hours.
- Ability to work as a contributing member of the multidisciplinary team.
- Ability to read, write and carry out directions.
- Ability to assemble, maintain and record data in an accurate record.
- Must strictly adhere to safety protocols to work with infectious specimens, chemicals and other hazards.
- Must be capable of producing accurate results under time constraints, multi-tasking, and performing in a fast-paced and changing environment.
- Ability to establish and maintain effective working relationships with other employees.
- Ability to work under pressure, communicate and present information.
- Ability to read, interpret, and apply clinic policies and procedures.
- Ability to identify problems, recommend solutions, organize and analyze information.
- Ability to establish priorities and coordinate work activities.
- Ability to work independently, be goal-directed and have strong organizational skills.

- Effectively multitask without compromising quality.
- Ability to communicate with individuals and small groups with credibility and confidence.
- Ability to handle difficult situations, remain calm under stress, manage emotional situations, display empathy and maintain positive communication during a rapidly changing/dynamic environment.
- Turn problems into opportunities by developing innovative and creative solutions.
- Demonstrate a friendly, positive attitude, display energy and drive in performing daily responsibilities.
- Must be flexible as well as easily adapt to a changing work environment which will require ongoing maintenance of job-related skills/activities.

Equipment Operated:

- Various and diverse healthcare equipment and machinery.
- Networked computer

Work Environment:

Position is in a well-lighted clinical environment.
Evening and weekend work.

Mental/Physical Requirements:

- Lifting—Not to exceed 50 lbs.—local practice may apply.
- Writing
- Sitting
- Standing spends majority of the shift working on their feet
- Bending
- Visual acuity
- Reading
- Field of vision/peripheral

- Regularly required to use hands to finger, handle, or feel objects, tools, or controls; bend, reach with hands and arms; stoop, kneel, and talk and/or hear.
- Noise
- Chemical vapors
- Infectious Materials

Disclaimer: This description is intended to provide only basic guidelines for meeting job requirements. Responsibilities, knowledge, skills, abilities, and working conditions may change as needs of the organization evolve and on an organization by organization basis.

Job Title: Labor and Delivery Nurse

Department: Obstetrics, Women's Health, or Clinical Services

Immediate Supervisor: Title: Manager of OB/GYN, Women's Health, or Clinical Services

Job Supervisory Responsibilities: None

General Summary:

A position responsible for providing prenatal education and support, attending childbirth, providing encouragement during labor and delivery, and supervising the general care of women and children directly after birth.

Provides care to women during normal pregnancies and deliveries and calls on obstetricians or other physicians if complications develop.

Essential Job Responsibilities:

- Performs the nursing duties related to midwifery including gynecological exams, preconception care, prenatal care, labor and delivery care, care after birth, newborn care, disease prevention, family planning, health maintenance counseling, and menopausal management.
- Enhance patient experiences; optimizing company reputation.
- Ensure compliance with current healthcare regulations, medical laws, federal and state laws, and high ethical standards.
- Maintain patient flow.
- Perform various patient care activities and related nonprofessional services necessary in personal needs and comforts of patients.
- Educates women about different types of care available and encourages them to enhance their pregnancy by being involved.

- Emphasizes patient education, active participation, clear communication between the provider and the woman, and an individualized health care experience.
- Advocates birth education, natural childbirth, and the participation of the entire family. Relies on technology only when medically necessary.
- Writes prescriptions as needed.
- Serves as OB/GYN team member working closely with physicians and other staff to ensure healthy pregnancies and deliveries.
- Provides emotional and social support, which can reduce the length of labor, the need for pain medication, the likelihood for use of forceps or other operative devices during delivery, or the possibility of cesarean delivery.
- Oversees the medical care of assigned pregnant patients under the supervision of a physician.
- Provides support to mother and family.
- Teaches patients about elements of mother–baby bonding, protecting from inadequate heat, overstimulation, noisy/brightly lit environments, cuddling/ hugging, recognizing signs of infant pain/ discomfort, and breast feeding.

Education:

- BSN.

Experience:

- Minimum three years of experience as RN; preferably in medical practice setting.

Other Requirements:

- Current RN state license.
- Current CPR certificate.
- Certification by state as a certified nurse midwife.

- Certification by ACNM, including meeting recommended ACNM continuing competency requirements and passing the national certification examination.

Competency Requirements:

Knowledge:

- Knowledge of nurse midwifery principles and techniques.
- Knowledge of methods ensuring safe working environment for patient, family, and staff including using appropriate personal protection equipment.
- Knowledge of theories of family dynamics, mother–child attachment, parenting, and adult learning concepts.

Skills:

- Skill in midwifery through appropriate prenatal education and support, coaching during pregnancy and delivery.
- Skill in showing parents how to use distraction techniques to calm baby, deal with sibling rivalry, practice effective parenting techniques.
- Skill in showing other staff how to best help pregnant/postpartum women by effective teaching of principles and methods.

Abilities:

- Ability to demonstrate full range of motion, eye–hand coordination, and manual/finger dexterity.
- Ability to assess a situation, consider alternatives, and choose an appropriate course of action.
- Ability to participate effectively as a team member.

Equipment Operated:

- Standard OB/GYN equipment for examining and caring for patient during pregnancy and delivery.

Work Environment:

Combination of office, exam, and birthing rooms.

Frequent exposure to communicable diseases, toxic substances, medicinal preparations, and other conditions common to a medical practice environment.

Mental/Physical Requirements:

- Varied activities including sitting, standing, walking, bending, reaching, and lifting.
- Occasionally lifts and carries items weighing up to 100 pounds.
- Stress related to dealing with anxious patients and responsibility for baby and mother.

Disclaimer: This description is intended to provide only basic guidelines for meeting job requirements. Responsibilities, knowledge, skills, abilities, and working conditions may change as needs of the organization evolve and on an organization by organization basis.

Job Title: Nutritionist
Department: Clinical Services
Immediate Supervisor Title: Clinical Services Manager
Job Supervisory Responsibilities: None

General Summary:

A position responsible for nutrition assessment, counseling, education, and program evaluation.

Essential Job Responsibilities:

- Assesses client medical history, including nutritional status, diet history, and food habits. Conducts individual sessions to discuss patient's nutritional needs and determine risk factors. Confers with physician and other clinicians as appropriate on effect of nutritional status.
- Develops nutritional plan for patient, presents information to patient/family individually about implementing nutrition plan including recommendations for special diets and diet techniques to ensure proper preparation and nutritional intake.
- Enhance patient experiences; optimizing company reputation.
- Ensure compliance with current healthcare regulations, medical laws, federal and state laws, and high ethical standards.
- Documents dietary assessment/plan summary for medical record.
- Conducts patient education programs for weight reduction, cultural preferences, and special-need diets for certain health conditions such as diabetes, high blood pressure, etc.

- Teaches correct food preparation and safe food handling. Conducts nutritional health education programs for staff.
- Acts as liaison with food access and subsidy programs.
- Participates collaboratively with other providers and resources to assess and address health issues including the development of community standards and programs.

Education:

- Bachelor's degree in nutrition, food service, or community health.
- Master's degree preferred.

Experience:

- Minimum three years of experience as dietitian.
- Two years of experience in health setting as dietitian/patient educator preferred.

Other Requirements:

- Registered dietitian as certified by the American Dietetic Association.

Competency Requirements:

Knowledge

- Knowledge of theoretical and practical principles related to nutrition and dietetics.
- Knowledge of medical terminology, universal precautions and food sanitation/safety procedures, and federal/state regulations related to food preparation, storage, etc.
- Knowledge of ethnic eating patterns and cultural customs related to food.

- Knowledge of education principles including human behavior and behavior modification techniques and presentation methods.

Skills:

- Skill in nutrition assessment.
- Skill in problem-solving and handling crisis situations.
- Skill in utilizing behavioral modification techniques to improve patient nutritional status.
- Skill in developing and presenting patient/staff/ community education workshops.

Abilities:

- Ability to read and follow written and oral medical orders.
- Ability to analyze medical condition and make appropriate judgments about dietary issues.
- Ability to work effectively in collaborative clinical and community situations. Equipment Operated: Standard office equipment, including computer.

Work Environment:

Combination of office, exam rooms, and classrooms.
May be exposed to communicable diseases and other conditions common to clinic setting.

Mental/Physical Requirements:

- Varied activities including sitting, walking, reaching, bending, and lifting.
- Must be able to stand two to four hours during educational sessions.
- Occasionally required to carry equipment and supplies weighing up to 50 pounds.
- Low level of stress.

Disclaimer: This description is intended to provide only basic guidelines for meeting job requirements. Responsibilities, knowledge, skills, abilities, and working conditions may change as needs of the organization evolve and on an organization by organization basis.

Job Title: Licensed Practical Nurse

Department: Patient Care

Immediate Supervisor Title: Physicians

Job Supervisory Responsibilities:

General Summary:

The Lead Licensed Practical Nurse - LPN is responsible for supervising nursing personnel to deliver nursing care and within scope of practice coordinates care delivery, which will ensure that patients needs are met in accordance with professional standards of practice through physician orders, center policies and procedures, and federal, state and local guidelines.

The Lead LPN position is a staff position that has direct care responsibilities as well as supervisor responsibility for nursing assistants.

Serve as an example to the LPN staff, provide direction in the absence of a supervisor.

Education:

- Graduate from an accredited school of practical nursing or vocational nursing.
- Valid state license to practice nursing.
- Current BLS certification.

Experience:

- One-year prior nursing experience preferred.

Other Requirements:

- Must be available to have a mixed schedule of opening and closing the office and the ability to be flexible with schedule when needed.

Competency requirements:

Knowledge:

- Knowledge of and experience with Epic is preferred
- Knowledge of proper phone etiquette and phone handling skills
- Knowledge of organizational policies, procedures, and systems.
- Knowledge of office management techniques and practices.
- Knowledge of computer systems, programs, and applications.
- Knowledge of research methods and procedures sufficient to compile data and prepare reports.
- Knowledge of grammar, spelling, and punctuation.
- General knowledge of healthcare terminology preferred.
- Knowledge of purchasing, budgeting, and inventory control.

Skills:

- Skill in taking and transcribing dictation and in the operation of office equipment.
- Ability to communicate in English, both verbally and in writing.
- Additional languages preferred.
- CPT & IDC9 coding abilities preferred.
- Requires strong personal computer skills, communication skills, problem solving, continuous improvement and teaming skills.
- Maintains a broad knowledge of clinical, financial, and administrative systems/applications and processes.
- Serves as a resource on department and institutional initiatives; shares knowledge with customers and colleagues.
- Demonstrated verbal and written communication skills.

Abilities:

- Must maintain regular and acceptable attendance; may be required to work weekend, holiday or OT hours.
- Ability to establish and maintain effective working relationships with other employees and the public.
- Ability to work under pressure, communicate and present information.
- Ability to read, interpret, and apply clinic policies and procedures.
- Ability to identify problems, recommend solutions, organize and analyze information.
- Ability to establish priorities and coordinate work activities.
- Exposure to electronic health record preferred.
- Ability to work independently, be goal-directed and have strong organizational skills.
- Effectively multitask without compromising quality.
- Ability to comprehend and excel in both verbal and written communication, including proper telephone etiquette, face-to-face interactions, and electronic communications.
- Ability to communicate with individuals and small groups with credibility and confidence.
- Ability to handle difficult situations, remain calm under stress, manage emotional situations, display empathy and maintain positive communication during a rapidly changing/dynamic environment.
- Turn problems into opportunities by developing innovative and creative solutions.
- Demonstrate a friendly, positive attitude, display energy and drive in performing daily responsibilities.
- Must be flexible as well as easily adapt to a changing work environment which will require ongoing maintenance of job-related skills/activities.
- Must be willing to adjust work schedules in response to department or clinical needs.

- Able to manage and prioritize tasks simultaneously while working directly with patients who may exhibit diverse needs.

Equipment Operated:

- Standard office equipment including computers, fax machines, copiers, printers, telephones, etc.

Work Environment:

Position is in a well-lighted office environment. Occasional evening and weekend work.

Mental/Physical Requirements:

- Lifting—Not to exceed 50 lbs.—local practice may apply.
- Writing , Sitting, Standing—spends majority of the shift working on their feet
- Bending Visual acuity, Reading
- Field of vision/peripheral
- Regularly required to use hands to finger, handle, or feel objects, tools, or controls; bend, reach with hands and arms; stoop, kneel, and talk and/or hear.
- Exposed to: Noise, Chemical vapors, Infectious Materials.
- Requires the ability to manage stressful situations.
- Occasional stress from varying demands.

Disclaimer: This description is intended to provide only basic guidelines for meeting job requirements. Responsibilities, knowledge, skills, abilities, and working conditions may change as needs of the organization evolve and on an organization by organization basis.

Job Title: LVN

Department: Nursing

Immediate Supervisor Title: Nursing Supervisor, Attending Physician

Job Supervisory Responsibilities:

General Summary:

Provides professional nursing care to clinic patients.

Works collaboratively with the providers within the team setting to facilitate quality care for the patient.

Essential Job Responsibilities:

- Performs general nursing care to patients.
- Administers treatments in accordance with nursing standards.
- Assists with the preparation of equipment and aids provider during treatment, examination, and testing of patients.
- Observes, records, and reports patients' condition and reaction to drugs or treatments to providers.
- Oversees appointment bookings and ensures preferences are given to patients in emergency situations. Maintains the timely flow of patients.
- Greets patients and obtains well-documented history and vitals.
- Prepares patients for a physical exam.
- Instructs patients in collection of samples and tests.
- May perform the following tasks in accordance with established procedures and as prescribed by applicable licensure/certification:
- Obtain/record vital signs; perform initial assessment on patient; coordinate patient transfer to hospital and/ or discharge; give telephone orders; accept telephone test results; perform telephone triage; call in provider approved prescription refills; specimen collection

including stool and urine midstream; catheterize patient; indwelling catheter urine collection; obtain throat culture; pregnancy testing; administer urine dip; obtain wound culture; perform Snellen vision screening; eye injury management; administer optic/optic meds; assist with lumbar punctures; sputum collection; occult blood testing; assist with vaginal exam; teach crutch/cane walking; teach use of walker; apply Velcro splint; assist with plaster splint; apply moist heat and/or cold packs; administer enema; remove fecal impaction; administer oxygen; teach respiratory hygiene; administer chest physiotherapy; perform oral suction and/or infant suction bulb; wound care; apply sterile dressing; assist with circumcision; perform umbilical care; apply colloidal dressing; open sterile tray; apply topical medications; administer rectal and/or vaginal medications; give oral medications; and, give sublingual medications to adults and/or pediatric patients.

- May perform the following tasks only if appropriate training has been obtained:
- Blood collection by lancet; pulse oximetry; incentive Spirometry; suture and/or staple removal; ear irrigation; administer breathing treatment; give allergy/insulin/immunization medications to adult and/or pediatric patients; give intramuscular and/or subcutaneous injections to adult and/or pediatric patients; give injections Z track to adult patients.
- May perform the following tasks after providing verification of completion of special training:
- Blood collection venipuncture; audiometry exam; Titmus vision screening; EKG; administer electrical stimulation; assist/process biopsies; draw blood from portocath; assist endoscopy, start saline lock or IV fluids and monitor IV fluids.

- May administer IV push medications and/or add medications to IV only after completion of special training and only under direct supervision of a licensed practitioner.
- May arrange for patient testing and admissions.
- May be required to have a working knowledge of ICD9, CPT and HCPCS coding and managed care.
- Respond to incoming telephone calls and (per provider instructions) calls in refills and prescriptions to the pharmacy.
- Per provider and/or established protocol, instructs patients and/or family with regard to medication and treatment and documents the same.
- Formulates and updates patient care plans. Orders, prepares, and inspects patient charts. Posts tests and examination results. Reviews patient's tests and examination results with the provider; documents instructions and notifies patient.
- Maintains patient files, records, and other information in a professional manner following policies and procedures regarding documentation.
- Ensures preparation of exam rooms including re-stocking of treatment areas.
- Attends required meetings and participates in committees as requested.
- Participates in professional development activities and maintains professional licensure and affiliations.
- Participates in a comprehensive and collaborative interdisciplinary approach to health care while promoting patient advocacy in nursing practice.
- Maintains competency in the performance of technical procedures and clinical assessment skills as required within the office setting and is able to function as a role model for all staff members.
- Promptly and correctly performs any treatments or screening tests as required by the physician, ensuring

the patient has an adequate understanding of the procedures to minimize anxiety or discomfort.

- Follows the guidelines related to the Health Insurance Portability and Accountability Act (HIPAA), designed to prevent or detect unauthorized disclosure of Protected Health Information (PHI).
- Maintains strict confidentiality.
- Uses oral and written communication skills to effectively convey ideas in a clear, positive manner that is consistent with the Mission.
- Maintains established policies, procedures, objectives, quality assurance, safety, environmental and infection control.
- Implements job responsibilities in a manner that is consistent with the Mission and Code of Ethics and supportive of cultural diversity objectives.
- Supports and adheres to Service Guarantee.

Education:
- Graduate from an accredited school of practical nursing or vocational nursing.
- Valid state license to practice nursing.
- Current BLS certification.

Experience:
- LVN medical office experience is required

Other Requirements:
- Must have sympathetic attitude toward the care of the ill.
- Must be available to have a mixed schedule of opening and closing the office and the ability to be flexible with schedule when needed.
- MGMA certification.

Competency requirements:

Knowledge

- Knowledge of laboratory functions, medical terminology, a background in science and 1-2 years medical experience is preferred, but not required.
- Previous experience or knowledge of computers and keyboarding, telephone operations and other office equipment desired.
- Ability to accurately read specimen labels and work with numbers to prevent mislabeling.
- Must be organized, able to prioritize and work in a fast-paced environment.
- Must possess good human relations skills and be able to communicate effectively both orally and in written form.
- Must be able to work independently as well as in a team environment.
- Must be able to accommodate scheduling adjustments, off-shifts, holiday, and weekend work assignments.
- Requires the ability to be attentive to details and to adhere to strict safety requirements for handling infectious agents.

Skills:

- Ability to communicate in English, both verbally and in writing.
- Additional languages preferred.
- Technical skills to effectively complete required professional documentation and correspondence.
- Must be able to work independently and in a team environment.
- Addressing and rectifying patient and/or staff concerns.
- High-level problem solving skills with flexible solutions for a changing healthcare market.
- Uses VMPS to identify a problem, route cause, and engages the team in solutions.

- Able to navigate through multiple electronic applications and devices, medical equipment, examples include iPad/tablets, Text Reminder notifications.

Abilities:

- Must maintain regular and acceptable attendance; may be required to work weekend, holiday or OT hours.
- Ability to work as a contributing member of the multidisciplinary team.
- Ability to read, write and carry out directions.
- Ability to assemble, maintain and record data in an accurate record.
- Must strictly adhere to safety protocols to work with infectious specimens, chemicals and other hazards.
- Must be capable of producing accurate results under time constraints, multi-tasking, and performing in a fast-paced and changing environment.
- **Ability to establish and maintain effective working relationships with other employees.**
- Ability to work under pressure, communicate and present information.
- Ability to read, interpret, and apply clinic policies and procedures.
- Ability to identify problems, recommend solutions, organize and analyze information.
- Ability to establish priorities and coordinate work activities.
- Ability to work independently, be goal-directed and have strong organizational skills.
- Effectively multitask without compromising quality.
- Ability to communicate with individuals and small groups with credibility and confidence.
- Ability to handle difficult situations, remain calm under stress, manage emotional situations, display empathy and maintain positive communication during a rapidly changing/dynamic environment.

- Turn problems into opportunities by developing innovative and creative solutions.
- Demonstrate a friendly, positive attitude, display energy and drive in performing daily responsibilities.
- Must be flexible as well as easily adapt to a changing work environment which will require ongoing maintenance of job-related skills/activities.

Equipment Operated:

- Various and diverse healthcare equipment and machinery.
- Networked computer

Work Environment:

Position is in a well-lighted clinical environment.
Occasional evening and weekend work.

Mental/Physical Requirements:

- Lifting—Not to exceed 50 lbs.
- Writing, Sitting, Bending, Visual acuity, Reading, Field of vision/peripheral
- Standing—spends majority of the shift working on their feet
- Regularly required to use hands to finger, handle, or feel objects, tools, or controls; bend, reach with hands and arms; stoop, kneel, and talk and/or hear.
- Exposure to: Noise, Chemical vapors, Infectious Materials
- Combination of sitting, standing, bending, light lifting and walking.
- Requires a full range of body motion including manual and finger dexterity and hand-eye coordination.
- Requires corrected vision and hearing to a normal range.
- Requires the ability to manage stressful situations.
- Occasional stress from varying demands.

Disclaimer: This description is intended to provide only basic guidelines for meeting job requirements. Responsibilities, knowledge, skills, abilities, and working conditions may change as needs of the organization evolve and on an organization by organization basis.

> **Job Title: Clinical Services Manager**
>
> **Department: Administration**
>
> **Immediate Supervisor Title: Practice Administrator**
>
> **Job Supervisory Responsibilities: Clinical staff**

General Summary:

The Clinical Services Manager supervises the Clinical Services Associates (CSA) assists the practice manager and physicians in maintaining a patient/customer focus, supports the delivery of high quality care, shares a passion for patient and customer centered care, and assists in meeting or exceeding patient satisfaction and financial/operational targets. The CSA supports the practice by performing clinical and administrative duties as a Medical Assistant and as a Patient Services Associate. The practice will determine, based on operational need, how much time will be spent in each capacity (MA and PSA).

Essential Job Responsibilities:

- Plans financial audits by understanding organization objectives, structure, policies, processes, internal controls, and external regulations; identifying risk areas; preparing audit scope and objectives; preparing audit programs.
- Assesses compliance with financial regulations and controls by executing audit program steps; testing general ledger, account balances, balance sheets, income statements, and related financial statements; examining and analyzing records, reports, operating practices, and documentation.
- Assesses risks and internal controls by identifying areas of non-compliance; evaluating manual and automated financial processes; identifying process weaknesses and inefficiencies and operational issues.

- Verifies assets and liabilities by comparing and analyzing items and collateral to documentation.
- Completes audit work papers and memoranda by documenting audit tests and findings.
- Communicates audit progress and findings by providing information in status meetings; highlighting unresolved issues; reviewing working papers; preparing final audit reports.
- Improves protection by recommending changes in management monitoring, assessment, and motivational practices, in the internal control structure, and in operating processes; identifying root causes.
- Supports external auditors by coordinating information requirements.
- Provides financial control information by collecting, analyzing, and summarizing data and trends.
- Protects organization's reputation by keeping information confidential.
- Updates job knowledge by participating in educational opportunities; reading professional publications; maintaining personal networks; participating in professional organizations.
- Contributes to team results by welcoming new and different work requirements; exploring new opportunities to add value to the organization; helping others accomplish related job results as and where needed.

Education:

- 2 or 4 year college degree required.
- Completion of an accredited Medical Assistant program required. .
- Minimum Certifications, Registry and/or Licenses Required:
- MA Certification required (required within 90 days of hire in certain geographic or complex specialty areas).

- CPR Certification required.

Experience:

- 2-3 years of CSA experience, or 4 years of customer service experience, required.
- Advanced degree (Associates, Bachelors, Masters) may be considered in lieu of experience.
- Thorough knowledge of third party insurance coverage guidelines preferred.

Other Requirements:

- Must be available to have a mixed schedule of opening and closing the office and the ability to be flexible with schedule when needed.
- MGMA certification.

Competency requirements:

Knowledge:

- Knowledge of organizational policies, procedures, and systems.
- Knowledge of office management techniques and practices.
- Knowledge of computer systems, programs, and applications.
- Knowledge of grammar, spelling, and punctuation.
- General knowledge of healthcare terminology preferred.
- Knowledge of purchasing, budgeting, and inventory control.

Skills:

- Ability to communicate in English, both verbally and in writing.
- Additional languages preferred.
- Must possess strong human relations, communication, problem solving, and organizational skills to interact

with a variety of customers and personnel, both within and outside the institution.

- Must be able to work independently and in a team environment.
- Requires strong personal computer skills, communication skills, problem solving, continuous improvement and teaming skills.
- Maintains a broad knowledge of clinical, financial, and administrative systems/applications and processes.
- Serves as a resource on department and institutional initiatives; shares knowledge with customers and colleagues.
- Demonstrated verbal and written communication skills.

Abilities:

- Must maintain regular and acceptable attendance; may be required to work weekend, holiday or OT hours.
- Ability to establish and maintain effective working relationships with other employees and the public.
- Ability to work under pressure, communicate and present information.
- Ability to read, interpret, and apply clinic policies and procedures.
- Ability to identify problems, recommend solutions, organize and analyze information.
- Ability to establish priorities and coordinate work activities.
- Exposure to electronic health record preferred.
- Ability to work independently, be goal-directed and have strong organizational skills.
- Effectively multitask without compromising quality.
- Ability to comprehend and excel in both verbal and written communication, including proper telephone etiquette, face-to-face interactions, and electronic communications.
- Ability to communicate with individuals and small groups with credibility and confidence.

- Ability to handle difficult situations, remain calm under stress, manage emotional situations, display empathy and maintain positive communication during a rapidly changing/dynamic environment.
- Turn problems into opportunities by developing innovative and creative solutions.
- Demonstrate a friendly, positive attitude, display energy and drive in performing daily responsibilities.
- Must be flexible as well as easily adapt to a changing work environment which will require ongoing maintenance of job-related skills/activities.
- Must be willing to adjust work schedules in response to department or clinical needs.
- Able to manage and prioritize tasks simultaneously while working directly with patients who may exhibit diverse needs.

Equipment Operated:

- Standard office equipment including computers, fax machines, copiers, printers, telephones, etc.

Work Environment:

Position is in a well-lighted office environment. Occasional evening and weekend work.

Mental/Physical Requirements:

- Involves sitting approximately 90 percent of the day, walking or standing the remainder.
- Combination of sitting, standing, bending, light lifting and walking.
- Requires a full range of body motion including manual and finger dexterity and hand-eye coordination.
- Requires corrected vision and hearing to a normal range.
- Requires the ability to manage stressful situations.
- Occasional stress from varying demands.

Disclaimer: This description is intended to provide only basic guidelines for meeting job requirements. Responsibilities, knowledge, skills, abilities, and working conditions may change as needs of the organization evolve and on an organization by organization basis.

Job Title: Occupational Therapist

Department: Rehabilitation Therapy Department or Clinical Services Department

Immediate Supervisor Title: Rehabilitation Therapy Manager or Clinical Services Manager

Job Supervisory Responsibilities: May participate in supervision of occupational therapy assistants

---

General Summary:

A position responsible for helping patients improve their ability to perform tasks in their daily living and working environments. Patients may have conditions that are mentally, physically, developmentally, or emotionally disabling.

Essential Job Responsibilities:

- Assesses patients and develops treatment plans in collaboration with physicians and other clinicians.
- Enhance patient experiences; optimizing company reputation.
- Ensure compliance with current healthcare regulations, medical laws, federal and state laws, and high ethical standards.
- Assists patients to develop, recover, or maintain daily living and work skills.
- Helps patients to improve their basic motor functions and reasoning ability and to compensate for any permanent loss of function to reach the goal of having independent, productive, and satisfying lives.
- Helps patients in performing a variety of activities from operating a computer to dealing with daily needs such as dressing, cooking, and eating.
- Assists patients with exercises that increase strength and dexterity, visual acuity, and the ability to discern patterns.

- Uses variety of equipment during treatment including computer programs to help patients improve decision making, abstract reasoning, problem solving, perceptual skills, memory, sequencing, and coordination to aid in independent living.
- Teaches patients, particularly those with permanent disabilities such as spinal cord injuries, cerebral palsy, or muscular dystrophy, in the use of adaptive equipment including wheelchairs, orthotics, and aids for eating and dressing.
- Follows medical practice policies related to compliance, safety, and infection control. Documents patient treatment and outcomes in medical record.

Education:

- Bachelor's degree in occupational therapy from accredited school plus master's degree in field.

Experience:

- Minimum two years of experience, preferably in clinic setting.

Other Requirements:

- Must have sympathetic attitude toward the care of the ill.
- Must be available to have a mixed schedule of opening and closing the office and the ability to be flexible with schedule when needed.
- MGMA certification.
- Current state occupational therapist license, successful completion of national certification examination.
- Current CPR certificate.

Competency requirements:

Knowledge:

- Knowledge of occupational therapy principles, standards, and applications.
- Knowledge of physical, biological, and behavioral sciences as well as application of occupational therapy equipment, devices, and patient-specific therapeutic devices. Understanding of how to modify equipment as needed.
- Knowledge of clinic policies and regulations related to infection control, safety, and quality improvement.

Skills:

- Skill in evaluating and treating patients.
- Skill in proper use of occupational therapy equipment and devices.
- Skill in assessing and recording patient activities and progress.

Abilities:

- Ability to collaborate with patients, families, and employers to modify workplace or home environment in line with patient's condition, including identification of environmental factors and hazards.
- Ability to communicate with patients and families in caring and compassionate manner to encourage behavioral changes.
- Ability to analyze patient data and behavior and modify treatment plan as appropriate.

Equipment Operated:

- Variety of therapeutic equipment including wheelchairs, orthotics, and aids for activities of daily living. Computer hardware and software for record keeping.

Work Environment:

Exam, treatment, and exercise rooms. May also occasionally require visits to patient homes and workplaces. Exposure to communicable diseases, biohazards, and conditions related to clinic setting.

Mental/Physical Requirements:

- Lifting—Not to exceed 50 lbs.
- Writing, Sitting, Bending, Visual acuity, Reading, Field of vision/peripheral
- Standing—spends majority of the shift working on their feet
- Regularly required to use hands to finger, handle, or feel objects, tools, or controls; bend, reach with hands and arms; stoop, kneel, and talk and/or hear.
- Exposure to: Noise, Chemical vapors, Infectious Materials
- Combination of sitting, standing, bending, light lifting and walking.
- Requires a full range of body motion including manual and finger dexterity and hand-eye coordination.
- Requires corrected vision and hearing to a normal range.
- Requires the ability to manage stressful situations.
- Occasional stress from medical situations.

Disclaimer: This description is intended to provide only basic guidelines for meeting job requirements. Responsibilities, knowledge, skills, abilities, and working conditions may change as needs of the organization evolve and on an organization by organization basis.

Job Title: Nursing Manager

Department: Nursing

Immediate Supervisor Title: Director of Nursing

Job Supervisory Responsibilities: Nurse supervisors.

General Summary:

The nurse manager 24/7 practice is accountable for the implementation of the vision, mission and values of Clinic and the Department of Nursing within defined areas of practice.

The nurse manager 24/7 practice plans, directs, coordinates, and evaluates the operational, fiscal, and personnel activities within defined areas of practice to ensure the provision of quality patient care 24 hours a day.

The individual contributes to the strategic planning process, and attainment of goals of the organization.

The individual is responsible for one or more inpatient units based upon unit/area complexity and size of practice.

The nurse manager 24/7 practice advocates for and allocates available resources to promote efficient, effective, safe, and compassionate nursing care based on current standards of practice.

The nurse manager 24/7 practice is responsible for total work unit budget.

The individual promotes shared decision making on the unit level.

The nurse manager 24/7 practice acts as a resource and facilitates collaboration between nursing personnel and other health care disciplines throughout the organization and within the healthcare community.

The nurse manager 24/7 is accountable for promoting ongoing development of all staff and for maintaining a professional environment in which all staff can grow and develop.

Direct reports may include nurse supervisors of assigned inpatient units.

Education:

- Graduate of an accredited baccalaureate nursing program.
- Maintains current Basic Life Support for Health Care Providers from one of the following programs: American Heart Associate or American Red Cross
- Graduate of an Accreditation Commission for Education in Nursing (ACEN)or Commission on Collegiate Nursing Education (CCNE)accredited
- Master's in Nursing or Doctor of Nursing Practice (DNP)program, business, or health related field as approved by Clinic Nurse Executive Committee preferred.
- Maintains ACLS and PALS per specific unit guidelines
- Any additional specialty certification/training as required by the work area.
- Current state RN license or current license deemed acceptable by the State Board of Nursing in which the RN practices.

Experience:

- Minimum of three years of nursing practice experience.
- Experience in the department's specialty preferred.
- Management experience preferred.

Other Requirements:

- Must have sympathetic attitude toward the care of the ill.
- Must be available to have a mixed schedule of opening and closing the office and the ability to be flexible with schedule when needed.
- MGMA certification.

Competency requirements:

Knowledge

149

- Knowledge of laboratory functions, medical terminology, a background in science and 1-2 years medical experience is preferred, but not required.
- Previous experience or knowledge of computers and keyboarding, telephone operations and other office equipment desired.
- Ability to accurately read specimen labels and work with numbers to prevent mislabeling.
- Must be organized, able to prioritize and work in a fast-paced environment.
- Must possess good human relations skills and be able to communicate effectively both orally and in written form.
- Must be able to work independently as well as in a team environment.
- Must be able to accommodate scheduling adjustments, off-shifts, holiday, and weekend work assignments.
- Requires the ability to be attentive to details and to adhere to strict safety requirements for handling infectious agents.

Skills:

- Ability to communicate in English, both verbally and in writing.
- Additional languages preferred.
- Must be able to work independently and in a team environment.
- Addressing and rectifying patient and/or staff concerns.
- High-level problem solving skills with flexible solutions for a changing healthcare market.
- Uses VMPS to identify a problem, route cause, and engages the team in solutions.
- Able to navigate through multiple electronic applications and devices, medical equipment, examples include iPad/tablets, Text Reminder notifications.

Abilities:

- Must maintain regular and acceptable attendance; may be required to work weekend, holiday or OT hours.
- Ability to read, write and carry out directions.
- Ability to assemble, maintain and record data in an accurate record.
- Must strictly adhere to safety protocols to work with infectious specimens, chemicals and other hazards.
- Must be capable of producing accurate results under time constraints, multi-tasking, and performing in a fast-paced and changing environment.
- **Ability to establish and maintain effective working relationships with other employees.**
- Ability to work under pressure, communicate and present information.
- Ability to read, interpret, and apply clinic policies and procedures.
- Ability to identify problems, recommend solutions, organize and analyze information.
- Ability to establish priorities and coordinate work activities.
- Ability to work independently, be goal-directed and have strong organizational skills.
- Effectively multitask without compromising quality.
- Ability to communicate with individuals and small groups with credibility and confidence.
- Ability to handle difficult situations, remain calm under stress, manage emotional situations, display empathy and maintain positive communication during a rapidly changing/dynamic environment.
- Turn problems into opportunities by developing innovative and creative solutions.
- Demonstrate a friendly, positive attitude, display energy and drive in performing daily responsibilities.
- Must be flexible as well as easily adapt to a changing work environment which will require ongoing maintenance of job-related skills/activities.

Equipment Operated:

- Various and diverse healthcare equipment and machinery.
- Networked computer

Work Environment:

Position is in a well-lighted clinical environment.
Occasional evening and weekend work.

Mental/Physical Requirements:

- Lifting—Not to exceed 50 lbs.
- Writing, Sitting, Bending, Visual acuity, Reading, Field of vision/peripheral
- Standing—spends majority of the shift working on their feet
- Regularly required to use hands to finger, handle, or feel objects, tools, or controls; bend, reach with hands and arms; stoop, kneel, and talk and/or hear.
- Exposure to: Noise, Chemical vapors, Infectious Materials
- Combination of sitting, standing, bending, light lifting and walking.
- Requires a full range of body motion including manual and finger dexterity and hand-eye coordination.
- Requires corrected vision and hearing to a normal range.
- Requires the ability to manage stressful situations.
- Occasional stress from medical situations.

Disclaimer: This description is intended to provide only basic guidelines for meeting job requirements. Responsibilities, knowledge, skills, abilities, and working conditions may change as needs of the organization evolve and on an organization by organization basis.

Job Title: Pharmacist
Department: Pharmacy
Immediate Supervisor Title: Pharmacy Manager
Job Supervisory Responsibilities: Pharmacy techs and staff

General Summary:

Responsibilities include distribution, drug therapy monitoring, education, and supervisory functions

Provides support to the Pharmacy and Therapeutics Committee, subcommittees, and workgroups.

Supports the continuous improvement, patient safety, and JCAHO accreditation programs of the department and institution.

Provides primary pharmacist coverage of the Drug Information Service.

Participates in educational and scholarly activities.

Enhance patient experiences; optimizing company reputation.

Ensure compliance with current healthcare regulations, medical laws, federal and state laws, and high ethical standards.

Provides support to other departmental functions and initiatives.

Detect, monitor, document, and report adverse drug reactions and medications errors.

Monitor drug therapy to evaluate appropriateness of use, dose, dosage form, regimen, route, therapeutic duplication, and drug interactions.

Communicate ongoing patient information, efficacy, and safety of treatment regimen(s) to all healthcare providers.

Education:

- Graduation from a Pharmacy program accredited by the Accreditation Council for Pharmacy Education.
- Doctor of Pharmacy (Pharm.D.) degree.

- Equivalent experience includes at least two years of relevant pharmacy practice experience.
- License to practice Pharmacy in the State.
- Current, active board certification in area of specialty

Experience:

- Completion of an accredited pharmacy residency.
- Experience in providing drug information within a formal Drug Information Services.
- Experience in quality monitoring and patient safety.
- History of scholarly activities including publication and scientific meeting presentations. Experience and / or interest in teaching.
- Prior experience in assigned area of specialty (e.g. Transplant, Infectious Disease, Hematology/Oncology) experience preferred.

Other Requirements:

- Must have sympathetic attitude toward the care of the ill.
- Must be available to have a mixed schedule of opening and closing the office and the ability to be flexible with schedule when needed.
- MGMA certification.

Competency Requirements:

Knowledge:

- Demonstrated knowledge of Pharmacist practices and principles.
- Demonstrated knowledge of Joint Commission, Federal and state regulations governing general Pharmacist practices and for acute care facilities.
- Must be organized, able to prioritize and work in a fast-paced environment.

- Must possess good human relations skills and be able to communicate effectively both orally and in written form.
- Must be able to work independently as well as in a team environment.
- Must be able to accommodate scheduling adjustments, off-shifts, holiday, and weekend work assignments.
- Requires the ability to be attentive to details and to adhere to strict safety.

Skills:

- Computer skills including internet, word processing, spreadsheet and data base applications. Project management and coordination skills.
- Commitment to excellence, accuracy, attention to detail and team work.
- Demonstrated skill in applying professional Pharmacy methods and techniques.
- Ability to communicate in English, both verbally and in writing.
- Additional languages preferred.
- Technical skills to effectively complete required professional documentation and correspondence.
- Addressing and rectifying patient and/or staff concerns.
- High-level problem solving skills with flexible solutions for a changing healthcare market.
- Uses VMPS to identify a problem, route cause, and engages the team in solutions.
- Able to navigate through multiple electronic applications and devices, medical equipment, examples include iPad/tablets, Text Reminder notifications.

Abilities:

- Ability to communicate effectively, works collaboratively with others, organizes time well, solve problems, and work independently with minimal supervision.

- The ability to assess data reflective of the patient's status and appropriately interpret information relative to the patient's age-specific needs is required.
- Must collaborate with others, organize well, accomplish tasks, solve problems, and communicate effectively.
- The individual must demonstrate knowledge of the principles of growth and development of the life span.
- The ability to assess data reflective of the patient's status and appropriately interpret information relative to the patient's age-specific needs is required.
- Demonstrated ability to communicate effectively both verbally and in writing to patients as well as other practitioners.
- Must be capable of producing accurate results under time constraints, multi-tasking, and performing in a fast-paced and changing environment.
- Ability to establish and maintain effective working relationships with other employees.
- Ability to work under pressure, communicate and present information.
- Ability to read, interpret, and apply clinic policies and procedures.
- Ability to identify problems, recommend solutions, organize and analyze information.
- Ability to establish priorities and coordinate work activities.
- Ability to work independently, be goal-directed and have strong organizational skills.
- Effectively multitask without compromising quality.
- Ability to communicate with individuals and small groups with credibility and confidence.
- Ability to handle difficult situations, remain calm under stress, manage emotional situations, display empathy and maintain positive communication during a rapidly changing/dynamic environment.

- Turn problems into opportunities by developing innovative and creative solutions.
- Demonstrate a friendly, positive attitude, display energy and drive in performing daily responsibilities.
- Must be flexible as well as easily adapt to a changing work environment which will require ongoing maintenance of job-related skills/activities.

Equipment Operated:

- Various and diverse healthcare equipment and machinery.
- Networked computer

Work Environment:

Position is in a well-lighted clinical environment.
Evening and weekend work.

Mental/Physical Requirements:

- Lifting—Not to exceed 50 lbs.—local practice may apply.
- Writing
- Sitting
- Standing—spends majority of the shift working on their feet
- Bending
- Visual acuity
- Reading
- Chemical vapors

Disclaimer: This description is intended to provide only basic guidelines for meeting job requirements. Responsibilities, knowledge, skills, abilities, and working conditions may change as needs of the organization evolve and on an organization by organization basis.

> ### Job Title: Physician Assistant
> ### Department: Patient Care
> ### Immediate Supervisor Title: Patient Care Director
> ### Job Supervisory Responsibilities: Nursing and Support Staff

General Summary:

A position responsible for practicing medicine with physician supervision including conducting examinations and writing prescriptions.

Within physician– physician assistant (PA) relationship, PAs exercise autonomy in medical decision making and provide a broad range of diagnostic and therapeutic services.

May practice in several primary care areas including family medicine, internal medicine, pediatrics, and obstetrics/gynecology as well as surgery and surgical subspecialties.

May include responsibility for education, research, and administrative services.

Essential Job Responsibilities:

- Conducts physical exams, assesses health status, orders and interprets tests, prescribes medications, and treats illnesses including giving injections and suturing wounds.
- Consults with physicians as needed and refers to physicians for more complicated medical cases or cases that are not a routine part of a PA's scope of work.
- Monitors therapies and provides continuity of care.
- Triages patient calls and evaluates patient problems. Responds to emergencies including use of CPR.
- Counsels patient/family on preventive health care.
- Documents patient information and care in medical record and may maintain department statistical database for research purposes.

- Enhance patient experiences; optimizing company reputation.
- Ensure compliance with current healthcare regulations, medical laws, federal and state laws, and high ethical standards.
- Maintain patient flow.

Education:

- Bachelor's degree and successful completion of accredited physician assistant program.

Experience:

- Four years of health care experience prior to applying to PA program, plus one year of experience as PA, preferably in clinic setting.

Other Requirements:

- National certification from the National Commission on Certification of PAs.
- To maintain their national certification, PAs must log 100 hours of continuing medical education every two years and sit for a recertification every six years.
- State PA license also required.
- Current CPR certificate required.

Competency Requirements:

Knowledge:

- Knowledge of medical model and roles of physicians and physician assistants. Familiar with anatomy, pharmacology, pathophysiology, clinical medicine, and physical diagnosis.
- Knowledge of patient assessment techniques including taking medical histories, performing physicals, evaluating health status including state of wellness, and compliance with care recommendations.
- Knowledge of diagnosing and treating medical problems and developing care plans.

- Knowledge of documentation in medical records in confidential manner.

Skills:

- Skill in gathering and analyzing physiological, socioeconomic, and emotional patient data.
- Skill in accurately evaluating patient problems in person or via phone and providing appropriate advice, intervention, or referral.
- Skill in developing/revising patient care plan based on patient status.

Abilities:

- Ability to make responsible decisions within scope of PA practice.
- Ability to collaborate effectively with physicians on complicated cases.
- Ability to educate patients, families, and staff in user-friendly manner.
- Ability to demonstrate eye–hand coordination, full range of motion, and manual dexterity.

Equipment Operated:

- Medical instruments required for physical exams and minor surgery and computer hardware/software.

Work Environment:

Medical office and exam room settings.
Frequent exposure to communicable diseases, biohazards, and other conditions common to clinic.
Frequent contact with variety of people.

Mental/Physical Requirements:

- Involves standing, sitting, walking, bending, stooping, and twisting.
- May be required to help to transfer patient.

- High level of responsibility and heavy workload can generate stress.

Disclaimer: This description is intended to provide only basic guidelines for meeting job requirements. Responsibilities, knowledge, skills, abilities, and working conditions may change as needs of the organization evolve and on an organization by organization basis.

Job Title: Nuclear Medicine Technologist

Department: Laboratory

Immediate Supervisor Title: Laboratory Manager

Job Supervisory Responsibilities:

General Summary:

A nonexempt position responsible for administering radiopharmaceuticals to patients for diagnostic purposes. May also perform radioimmunoassay studies.

Essential Job Responsibilities:

- Explains test procedures to patients and prepares dosages of radio-pharmaceuticals.
- Administers radiopharmaceuticals to patients by mouth, injection, inhalation, or other means. Positions patients on table or special chair.
- Adheres to safety standards that keep the radiation dose to patients and workers as low as possible.
- Starts a gamma scintillation camera, or scanner, which creates images of the distribution of a radiopharmaceutical as it localizes in, and emits signals from, the patient's body.
- Operates the camera to detect and map the radioactive drug in the patient's body to create diagnostic images.
- Monitors the characteristics and functions of tissues or organs in which the drugs localize to determine the presence of disease on the basis of biological changes rather than changes in organ structure.
- Produces the images on a computer screen or on film for a physician to interpret.
- Keeps patient records and records the amount and type of radionuclides received, used, and discarded.

- Performs radioimmunoassay computerized studies as requested that assess the behavior of a radioactive substance inside the body to determine levels of hormones or of therapeutic drugs in the body.

Education:

- High school diploma.
- Successful completion of nuclear medicine technology program leading to an associate's or bachelor's degree.

Experience:

- Minimum two years of experience as nuclear medicine technician, preferably in medical practice setting.

Other Requirements:

- Must be available to have a mixed schedule of opening and closing the office and the ability to be flexible with schedule when needed.
- MGMA certification.
- Most states require certification or licensure. Certification is available from the American Registry of Radiologic Technologists and from the Nuclear Medicine Technology Certification Board.

Competency requirements:

Knowledge:

- Knowledge of the physical sciences, biological effects of radiation exposure, radiation protection and procedures.
- Knowledge of radiopharmaceuticals, imaging techniques, and computer applications.
- Knowledge of safety, infection control, quality assurance, and confidentiality regulations.

Skills:

- Skill in sensitively understanding patients' physical and psychological needs.
- Skill in paying attention to details and in following instructions.
- Skill in administering radiopharmaceuticals and in operating camera and computer for imaging.

Abilities:

- Ability to explain the procedure to patients in calm, accurate manner.
- Ability to position patient and operate equipment effectively using mechanical abilities and manual dexterity.
- Ability to interact effectively with physicians and other clinicians as a team member.

Equipment Operated:

- Standard office equipment including computers, fax machines, copiers, printers, telephones, etc.
- Imaging equipment including cameras and computers. Special tables/chairs for positioning patients. Safety equipment including shielded syringes, gloves, and other protective devices. Technologists wear badges that measure radiation levels.

Work Environment:

Position is in a well-lighted clinic environment.

Occasional evening and weekend work.

Potential for radiation exposure is minimal because of safety precautions.

Some exposure to communicable diseases and other conditions related to medical environment.

Mental/Physical Requirements:

- Physical stamina needed because technologists are on their feet much of the day and may lift or turn disabled patients.
- May be required to lift/turn up to 100+ pounds.
- Stress related to dealing with anxious patients and need to be accurate and safe.
- Triage Telephone Nurse

Disclaimer: This description is intended to provide only basic guidelines for meeting job requirements. Responsibilities, knowledge, skills, abilities, and working conditions may change as needs of the organization evolve and on an organization by organization basis.

Job Title: Triage Telephone Nurse

Department: Clinical Services

Immediate Supervisor Title: Clinical Services Manager

Job Supervisory Responsibilities: None

General Summary:

An exempt position responsible for providing triage (sorting/ prioritizing patients) telephone service to ensure prompt identification of patients with high-risk conditions. May outsource this service to contractor.

Essential Job Responsibilities:

- Talks directly to patients on the telephone and then directs them to emergency rooms (ERs) or urgent care centers or to see their physician during office hours.

- Performs short evaluation of the patient situation to estimate severity of illness and/or injury including learning about chief complaint and, as possible, obtaining vital sign and mental status information.

- Determines urgency of seeing the patient based on brief assessment and on familiarity with a patient's condition and history. May use computerized medical information database, which uses algorithms that closely imitate physician logic and thought patterns, as guide. Confers with physician as needed.

- Sends those with high-risk chief complaints such as chest pain, abdominal pain, or severe headaches to ER immediately or arranges for ambulance. May provide appropriate home health advice to those patients who do not need to go directly to the ER.

- Sets up appointment for patients who do not need to go to ER but need to see a physician or arranges for an appointment scheduler to make the appointment.

- Acts, when designated, in "Ask a Nurse" capacity, handling routine information requests from patients, e.g., "Do I need a flu shot every year? When are you giving these shots?"

Education:

- RN degree; BSN or MSN degree preferred. On-the-job training in triage.

Experience:

- Minimum five years of experience as RN; one to two years of telephone triage experience, preferably in medical practice setting.

Other Requirements:

- Current state RN license. Current CPR certificate.

Competency requirements:

Knowledge:

- Knowledge of telephone-based clinical assessment techniques.
- Knowledge of medical practice telephone triage protocols.
- Knowledge of appropriate home health information for patients to follow until visit with physician, if they do not need an immediate ER visit.

Skills:

- Skill in using electronic medical records to check patient history.
- Skill in using computerized medical information database during evaluation as guide to appropriate decision.
- Skill in making triage decisions and responding quickly and calmly in emergency situations such as calling 911 and arranging for ambulance.

Abilities:

- Ability to communicate clearly and calmly with patient.
- Ability to elicit information needed to make brief evaluation.
- Ability to work closely with physicians and other clinicians as needed.

Equipment Operated:

- Telephone system at medical practice or contractor office. Computer hardware/ software for access to patient history and medical information databases.

Work Environment:

Office setting, well lighted, good air quality. Rare direct contact with patients.

Mental/Physical Requirements:

- Mostly sedentary position. Hand/arm injury possible from repetitive movements. Stress generated if high volume of calls and emergencies.

Disclaimer: This description is intended to provide only basic guidelines for meeting job requirements. Responsibilities, knowledge, skills, abilities, and working conditions may change as needs of the organization evolve and on an organization by organization basis.

Job Title: Radiation Therapist

Department: Laboratory

Immediate Supervisor Title: Laboratory Manager

Job Supervisory Responsibilities:

General Summary:

A position responsible for administering radiation treatment to patients under the direction of a radiation oncologist.

Essential Job Responsibilities:

- Prepares exam room and equipment. Explains procedure to patient. Takes medical history information if needed.
- Enhance patient experiences; optimizing company reputation.
- Ensure compliance with current healthcare regulations, medical laws, federal and state laws, and high ethical standards.
- Maintain patient flow.
- Uses an X-ray imaging machine to pinpoint the location of the tumor and/or computerized tomography (CT) scan to help determine how best to direct the radiation to minimize damage to healthy tissue.
- Positions patient and adjusts the linear accelerator to concentrate radiation exposure on the tumor cells following the treatment plan developed in conjunction with radiation oncologist. Explains procedure to the patient.
- Performs dosimetry procedures.
- Delivers accurately the prescribed planned course of radiation therapy.
- Monitors patient's physical condition during treatment phase to determine any adverse side effects.

- Documents all pertinent information in medical record including dose of radiation used for each treatment, total amount of radiation used to date, area treated, and patient's reactions.
- Performs daily linear accelerator warm-up procedures.
- Checks photon beam and all electron beams for consistency.
- Checks physics components for accuracy of beam alignment.
- Cares for brachytherapy sources including preparing for use, cleaning and returning to safe, keeping log of use.
- Follows radiation safety protocols in competent manner.

Education:

- Successful completion of an associate's or bachelor's degree program in radiation therapy or a radiography program, plus a 12-month certificate program in radiation therapy.

Experience:

- Minimum two years of experience as staff radiation therapist in radiation center, preferably in clinic setting.

Other Requirements:

- Must be available to have a mixed schedule of opening and closing the office and the ability to be flexible with schedule when needed.
- MGMA certification.
- Some states require state license. Also required by some states and employers is certification by the American Registry of Radiologic Technologists.

Competency Requirements:

Knowledge:

- Knowledge of radiation therapy theory and applications.

- Knowledge of radiation safety protocols.
- Knowledge of dosimetry and treatment planning.

Skills:

- Skill in effectively performing radiation procedures, particularly safety procedures.
- Skill in explaining radiation plans and treatments to patients and their families.
- Skill in identifying unsatisfactory set-up situations and/or errors and reporting them to radiation oncologist.

Abilities:

- Ability to observe and deal competently and compassionately with patient's emotional condition, maintaining a positive attitude and providing emotional support.
- Ability to collaborate effectively with health care team.
- Ability to demonstrate manual/finger dexterity, eye–hand coordination, and agility for use with equipment.

Equipment Operated:

- Standard office equipment including computers, fax machines, copiers, printers, telephones, etc.
- Radiation equipment and related items such as treatment table. Computer hardware and software for documentation purposes.

Work Environment:

Medical offices and exam rooms.
Clean, well lit, and well ventilated.
Exposure to radioactive materials and communicable diseases.

Mental/Physical Requirements:

- Considerable standing (four to six hours per day), walking, sitting, and stooping.

- May need to help transfer patients and lift/carry equipment weighing 75+ pounds.
- Stress related to need for safety and accuracy and dealing with anxious patients.

Disclaimer: This description is intended to provide only basic guidelines for meeting job requirements. Responsibilities, knowledge, skills, abilities, and working conditions may change as needs of the organization evolve and on an organization by organization basis.

Job Title: Optician

Department: Optical or Clinical Services
Immediate Supervisor Title: Optical Manager,
Optometrist, or Clinical Services Manager
Supervisory Responsibilities: May supervise optical technicians

General Summary

A medical position responsible for dispensing eyeglasses and contact lenses, following prescriptions written by ophthalmologists or optometrists.

Essential Job Responsibilities:

- Examines written prescriptions to determine the specifications of lenses.
- Recommends eyeglass frames, lenses, and lens coatings or contact lenses after considering the prescription and the patient's occupation, habits, and facial features.
- Measures patients' eyes, including the distance between the centers of the pupils and the distance between the ocular surface and the lens. Selects the type of contact lens material if this type of corrective device is chosen.
- Enhance patient experiences; optimizing company reputation.
- Ensure compliance with current healthcare regulations, medical laws, federal and state laws, and high ethical standards.
- Maintain patient flow.
- Perform various patient care activities and related nonprofessional services necessary in personal needs and comforts of patients.
- Set an example for and reinforcing evidence-based practices.
- Duplicates eyeglasses by using a focimeter to record eyeglass measurements. May obtain patient's previous

record in order to re-make eyeglasses or contact lenses or may verify prescription with the examining optometrist or ophthalmologist.

- Prepares work orders, including prescriptions for eyeglass lenses and information on their size, material, color, and style that give ophthalmic laboratory technician the information needed to grind and insert lenses into a frame. Prepares work order for contact lenses with similar information.
- Verifies that the lenses have been ground to specifications. May reshape or bend the eyeglass frame by hand or by using pliers so that the eyeglasses fit the patient properly and comfortably. May fix, adjust, and refit broken frames.
- Instructs patients about adapting to, wearing, and caring for eyeglasses. Instructs, often during several visits, patients on inserting, removing, and caring for contacts.
- Documents patient care and treatment. Follows safety, infection control, and quality assurance protocols.

Education:
- College or postsecondary optical training preferred.
- On-the-job training or two- to four-year apprenticeships often provided.

Experience:
- Minimum three years of clinical experience, preferably in optical laboratory or department.

Other Requirements:
- Some states require that dispensing opticians be licensed.
- Some states also may require applicants to pass a state practical exam, state written exam, or certification

exam offered by the American Board of Opticianry and the National Contact Lens Examiners.

- Willingness to work with underprivileged populations.
- Must have sympathetic attitude toward the care of the ill.
- Must be available to have a mixed schedule of opening and closing the office and the ability to be flexible with schedule when needed.
- MGMA certification.
- Satisfactory completion of background checking process.
- Willingness to adhere to stated program and documentation protocols.

Competency Requirements:

Knowledge:

- Knowledge of physics, basic anatomy, algebra, and trigonometry.
- Knowledge of optical equipment and instruments.
- Knowledge of safety, infection control, documentation, and quality improvement protocols.
- Ability to accurately read specimen labels and work with numbers to prevent mislabeling.
- Must be organized, able to prioritize and work in a fast-paced environment.
- Must possess good human relations skills and be able to communicate effectively both orally and in written form.
- Must be able to work independently as well as in a team environment.
- Must be able to accommodate scheduling adjustments, off-shifts, holiday, and weekend work assignments.

Skills:

- Skill in using computers for optical mathematics and optical physics.

- Skill in using precision measuring instruments and other optical machinery and tools.
- Skill in adjusting eyeglasses/contact lenses to best fit patients.
- Ability to communicate in English, both verbally and in writing.
- Additional languages preferred.
- Technical skills to effectively complete required professional documentation and correspondence.
- Addressing and rectifying patient and/or staff concerns.

Abilities:

- Ability to follow prescriptions and patient information to develop accurate work orders for ophthalmic lab technicians to make eyeglasses and contact lenses.
- Ability to collaborate effectively with optical clinical team.
- Ability to demonstrate eye–hand coordination, manual/finger dexterity, agility, and color vision and depth perception with visual acuity correctable to 20/25 while fitting eyeglasses and contacts.
- Ability to read, write and carry out directions.
- Ability to assemble, maintain and record data in an accurate record.
- Must strictly adhere to safety protocols to work with infectious specimens, chemicals and other hazards.
- Must be capable of producing accurate results under time constraints, multi-tasking, and performing in a fast-paced and changing environment.
- Ability to establish and maintain effective working relationships with other employees.
- Ability to work under pressure, communicate and present information.
- Ability to read, interpret, and apply clinic policies and procedures.
- Ability to identify problems, recommend solutions, organize and analyze information.

Equipment Operated:

- Variety of optical equipment and instruments including focimeters, pliers, and computer hardware/software.

Work Environment:

Medical office, exam and laboratory setting. Well-lighted and well-ventilated surroundings.

May be exposed to communicable diseases and other conditions related to clinic setting.

Mental/Physical Requirements:

- Combination of standing, sitting, walking, stooping, bending, and reaching.
- Occasionally must lift/carry up to 50 pounds.
- Low level of stress.
- Regularly required to use hands to finger, handle, or feel objects, tools, or controls; bend, reach with hands and arms; stoop, kneel, and talk and/or hear.

Disclaimer: This description is intended to provide only basic guidelines for meeting job requirements. Responsibilities, knowledge, skills, abilities, and working conditions may change as needs of the organization evolve and on an organization by organization basis.

Job Title: Patient Representative/Advocate

Department: Clinical Services

Immediate Supervisor Title: Clinical Services Manager

Job Supervisory Responsibilities:

General Summary:

A clinical position responsible for working directly with patients and their families to discuss any questions, complaints, comments, or suggestions.

Advocates for patient in resolution of concerns.

Essential Job Responsibilities:

- Enhance patient experiences; optimizing company reputation.
- Ensure compliance with current healthcare regulations, medical laws, federal and state laws, and high ethical standards.
- Serves as the clinic contact to resolve patient/family concerns and complaints.
- Gathers and researches appropriate information related to patient care, reimbursement, or community resource issues.
- Follows complaint through to resolution and provides feedback to patient/family. Facilitates relationships with public.
- Works with staff to resolve concerns and improve services, taking advocacy position.
- Tracks and analyzes all concerns and complaints. Identifies problematic trends and makes recommendations for correction.
- Produces regular overview reports.
- Develops referral systems with human services agencies and collaborates with community resource network.

Education:

- Bachelor's degree in human relations/social services, communications, marketing, or business/health administration.

Experience:

- Minimum two years of experience in customer services, with at least six months of experience in health care setting.
- Patient representative experience preferred.

Other Requirements:

- Must be available to have a mixed schedule of opening and closing the office and the ability to be flexible with schedule when needed.
- MGMA certification.

Competency requirements:

Knowledge:

- Knowledge of health care field; medical practice clinical and administrative systems, departments, and practices, including clinic financial policies and reimbursement payment requirements.
- Knowledge of counseling, conflict resolution, and customer service principles and applications.
- Knowledge of research methods to identify issues and clarify policies. Understanding of medical terminology. Familiarity with community resources.

Skills:

- Skill in analyzing data, policies, and requirements and in preparing objective,
- comprehensive reports using computers for both research and reporting.
- Skill in defusing tense situations through diplomatic problem-solving.

- Skill in effectively balancing needs of clinic with needs of patient with minimum of tension.

Abilities:

- Ability to communicate effectively with patients, staff, and external contacts via phone, in person, and through well-written reports.
- Ability to demonstrate leadership within medical practice to resolve immediate and long-term patient concerns.
- Ability to establish/maintain effective relationships with a wide variety of people.

Equipment Operated:

- Standard office equipment including computers, fax machines, copiers, printers, telephones, etc.

Work Environment:

- Position is in a well-lighted clinic environment.
- Occasional evening and weekend work.
- Some travel within the community.
- Constant contact with individuals from many backgrounds.
- Minimum exposure to communicable diseases.
- Frequent stress from dealing with tense individuals in uncomfortable situations.

Mental/Physical Requirements:

- Involves sitting approximately 90 percent of the day, walking or standing the remainder.
- Combination of sitting, standing, bending, light lifting and walking.
- Requires a full range of body motion including manual and finger dexterity and hand-eye coordination.
- Lifting up to 20 pounds.

- Requires corrected vision and hearing to a normal range.
- Requires the ability to manage stressful situations.
- Occasional stress from varying demands.
- Occasional stress from dealing with complex patient advocacy issues.
-

Disclaimer: This description is intended to provide only basic guidelines for meeting job requirements. Responsibilities, knowledge, skills, abilities, and working conditions may change as needs of the organization evolve and on an organization by organization basis.

Appendix B:
Sample Interview Questions

These are specific behavior-based questions for the different roles in patient access. Build on these to obtain the information needed to determine if the candidate has the skillset and abilities to address some of these common issues.

Standard Questions for Clinical Positions

There are many specific questions for each job title, this is a sampling of questions that could work for the above job titles in this category.

- How do you handle conflict in the workplace? Have you had situations in your past when you disagreed with your supervisor and how did you handle it?
- Do you have an elevator pitch? What's the biggest challenge in your role? How do you know you're successful?
- Customer Service (any role though)—Tell me about a time when you weren't successful in providing good

customer service. What did you learn and what would you do differently?
- Success—how do you know when you've been successful in your role?
- How do you explain what you do to a 5-year old?
- You're talking with a coworker/patient/customer/et al. and you notice a mistake on your materials, how do you handle this? What do you say?

Specific Questions for Clinical Positions

- **Nurse Manager/Director of Nursing**
  o How do you manage all of the pulling and pushing that goes on within a practice?
  o You're responsible for many aspects of the practice from patient satisfaction to employee challenges, how do you know you're successful in these areas?
  o Tell me about how you handle conflict with the practice owner or physicians.
  o How do you stay up to date on new techniques or care delivery models?
- **Team Leader**
  o Walk me through your background and what makes this role enticing
  o How would you refine our strategy to be more in line with the community and our competition?
  o Tell me about how you handle conflict with the management team.
  o Tell me about your past successes that you're proud of in your past roles
- **Audiologist**
  o What made you want to become an audiologist?
  o Walk me through a particularly difficult patient you've worked with in the past. How did you handle the difficult situation and what did you learn from it?

- How do you provide compassionate, empathetic care to your patients?
- Providing family and patient education is important, what do you always want to get across to them?

- **Certified Medical Assistant, Certified Nursing Assistant, Nurses' Aide**
  - You've picked a very difficult job, what do you find the most difficult about it? What do you like about it?
  - Walk me through a particularly difficult patient you've worked with in the past. How did you handle the difficult situation and what did you learn from it?
  - Have you experienced any negative outcomes with your patients? What was it and what happened?
  - How do you communicate with patients who do not speak your language or have special needs?

- **Clinical Staff Educator**
  - Providing education to employees is a difficult position. How do you approach new trainings to get the most out of the time with the employee?
  - Walk me through a time when you had staff who were not interested in learning. How did you handle this?
  - What is your experience with designing training materials?
  - How often do you update training materials?
  - How do you work with adult learners to get the best out of them?

- **Dialysis/Nephrology Nurse**
  - What are the top three things you monitor when providing hemodialysis, peritoneal dialysis and aphresis treatments?
  - What safety checks do you perform prior to providing services?

- How do you teach patients/families about the disease and the treatment plan?
- What irregular reactions do you notify the nephrologist?

- **EEG/EKG Technician**
  - Walk me through how you explain to the patient what you are doing.
  - What types of EMRs have you used previously?
  - What would you do with a malfunctioning unit? How do you handle if you're with a patient?
  - Have you experienced critical deviations in patient conditions? Walk me through what you did and how you handled.

- **Health Educator**
  - Have you developed patient educational materials in the past? If no - how would you go about doing that in the future? If yes—what did you create and how was it used?
  - How do you track information to report for quality measures on the education provided?
  - When working with patients who require different learning techniques, what do you do?
  - Share with me a patient experience that you feel was a particularly successful one thanks to the education you provided. Share a negative one.

- **Interpretive Services Coordinator**
  - Have you started a program from scratch?
  - Tell me how you would implement this program in our practice.

- **Laboratory Manager**
  - What does it mean when I say you'll supervise lab operations to maintain quality and efficiency?
  - How do you oversee training of staff? What types of training are essential?
  - What are ISO 17025 guidelines?

○ Tell me about a particularly great employee you've worked with in the lab previously.

- **Laboratory Technician**
  ○ Walk me through a typical procedure for specimen collection, handling and processing.
  ○ How do you distribute laboratory stock?
  ○ Documenting quality control activities is essential, what is your typical protocol for this?
  ○ How have you made a contribution to your past employers?

- **Licensed Practical Nurse (how come there isn't an LVN job title)**
  ○ How do you describe a compassionate nurse?
  ○ What do you think the difficulty is with families involved at bedside or in the care of the loved ones?
  ○ How do you handle patients who do not speak English?
  ○ Describe yourself in your nursing role.
  ○ Tell me about a time you disagreed with a treatment plan.

- **Mammographer/Mammography Technologist**
  ○ Walk me through the information you would give to a patient as you are providing the exam.
  ○ When have you been uncomfortable in this position?
  ○ Have you experienced difficult situations in the workplace while providing care?
  ○ What type of environment do you want to work in?
  ○ How do you know you're successful in this role?

- **Medical Manager/Clinical Services Manager**
  ○ As the manager, you have to give directions and sometimes negative information to the employees, walk me through how you approach this.
  ○ Implementing new techniques or programs can be challenging for the manager, how would you begin such an implementation?

- How do you handle the constant changes in healthcare?
- What makes you want to be the clinical manager as opposed to the care provider?

- **Nuclear Medicine Technologist**
  - Part of the responsibility of maintaining records of radioactive materials falls to the technologist. How do you maintain these records? What happens if the records are not maintained?
  - What types of communication do you use when doing your position? How can you comfort patients when they are stressed by this type of testing?
  - Walk me through recognizing possible adverse outcomes during the procedure.

- **Nurse Anesthetist**
  - How do you stay informed of changes in the industry or advancements in this role?
  - Working on a multidisciplinary team is essential, tell me about a difficult time you may have had with a staff member and how did it resolve?
  - Emergency situations arise in this role, how do you handle these types of situations?
  - Tell me about how you rate your interpersonal skills and what you think you need to improve upon.

- **Nurse Midwife**
  - Tell me about why you became a nurse midwife.
  - How do you handle the bad days in this role?
  - What do you think will set you apart from others as you interview for this role?
  - How do you keep abreast of changes and new ideas/concepts?
  - Share with me about a particularly successful outcome you've experienced.

- **Nurse Practitioner**
  - Have you dealt with physicians who aren't interested in collaborating? How has that played out? What would you do differently?
  - What types of communications methods do you employ to communicate with the physicians?
  - What types of patients do you have a passion for?
  - Share with me about a negative outcome that you were involved in.

- **Nutritionist**
  - As you meet with patients/families, I'm sure you've encountered some who aren't interested in changing their ways. How do you communicate with those types of patients?
  - When providing education, how do you handle the adult learner?
  - What techniques do you employ to work within the multidisciplinary team?
  - Overview your educational classes that you've provided to clients/patients? How would you implement a new training calendar for patients?

- **Occupational Therapist, Speech Language Pathologist/Therapist, Occupational Therapy Assistant, Physical Therapist/Physical Therapist Assistant**
  - When you have a patient who will benefit from services, but the services are limited, how do you handle this?
  - What is progress to you?
  - Tell me about a time when you had a particularly difficult patient, how did you handle this.
  - What do you have to learn as an OT, SLPT?
  - How do you stay abreast of new techniques and therapies in your field?

- **Oncology Nurse**
  - This is a position that requires a high level of compassion and caring. How do you do that on a daily basis and with difficult patients?
  - What one thing do you wish you knew before you entered this field?
  - Tell me about a particularly difficult patient you've worked with
  - Share the positive side of this position
  - When I say "must have great counseling skills"— what does that mean?
  - How do you evaluate effectiveness in patient care?
- **Optician**
  - Appearance of the facility/area is very important. How do you asses our optical rooms?
  - What would you change?
  - Why do you think this role is important here?
  - Glasses choosing, the process of this, is very personal. How do you help a client but not interfere?
- **Patient Representative/Advocate**
  - Part of this role that is vital is maintaining a positive outlook and disposition. How do you do that in this tough role?
  - Making a great first impression in this role is essential. What would you do to provide that?
  - When you disagree with the conversation or the methods to provide care, how do you handle this situation?
  - Have you been in a situation where you disagreed with the family or the patient's care plan? What did you do?
- **Pharmacist**
  - How do you review drug/drug interactions while managing patient meds?
  - Walk me through your process of handling interns or techs to assure accuracy and correct dispensing.

- ○ What types of policies or processes have you implemented previously to assure regularly compliance?
- **Phlebotomist**
  - ○ Walk me through how you welcome a patient in to the room.
  - ○ Describe the first and the last thing you do to the patient.
  - ○ What other roles are you interested in in the medical field?
  - ○ A patient complains that you are rough, what do you do?
  - ○ Have you received any patient complaints? What about compliments? Describe them to me.
- **Psychologist**
  - ○ Positive face-to-face interactions are essential in this role. Have you experienced a situation when you did not have a positive interaction? Walk me through what happened and how you handled it.
  - ○ Radiation Therapist
  - ○ As the therapist, you see patients at their most vulnerable. How do you handle the emotional spend it takes to do this?
  - ○ What types of computer systems have you used to document?
  - ○ What types of unusual reactions have you witnessed? How do you report to the physician?
  - ○ What does the team integrated approach mean to you?
- **Registered Nurse**
  - ○ How do you describe a compassionate nurse?
  - ○ What do you think the difficulty is with families involved at bedside or in the care of the loved ones?
  - ○ How do you handle patients who do not speak English?
  - ○ Describe yourself in your nursing role.

   o   Tell me about a time you disagreed with a treatment plan.
- **Respiratory Therapist**
   o   Walk me through how you incorporate quality improvement measurements in your work.
   o   How would you prioritize needs for the patient? How do you educate and coach the patient?
   o   Reporting therapeutic outcomes is a part of this position, what metrics will oyu be reviewing and looking at ongoing?
   o   Tell me about a time when you had a particularly difficult patient.
- **Social Worker**
   o   When you were in school, why did you decide to be a social worker?
   o   What is the hardest thing you do as a social worker?
   o   Tell me about a great success you had dealing with patients.
   o   Social workers have some of the hardest jobs. You see the difficulty for patients that they have in their everyday lives. How do you handle the stress and pressure when you go home?
- **Sonographer/ultra-sonographer**
   o   How do you provide information to the patient without acting like the physician?
   o   Walk me through how you would monitor the patient's well-being during the exam?
   o   Have you ever disagreed with the radiologist/ physician's results/assessment? How did you handle this?
   o   What makes you good at your job?
- **Surgical/Operating Technologist**
   o   This role is a conductor for the surgical needs. How do you maintain the accuacy and the precision in the room?

- o Constant maintenance of sterile equipment is to be maintained. Walk me through how you do that.
- o How do you stay up-to-date on new surgical processes and techniques?
- o What is enjoyable about this position?
- o As the technologies, you act as the primary person, how do you anticipate the needs of the physician?

- **Telemonitoring Nurse**
  - o Walk me through how you've monitored in the past? What equipment? How did you document and asses?
  - o What part of this role is interesting to you? What is not?
  - o Share with me a particularly difficult case you've had at work.

- **Triage Telephone Nurse**
  - o What type of systems have you usd in the past?

About the Authors

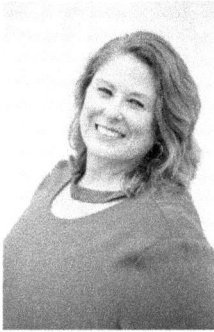

Penny M. Crow, MS, SHRM-SCP, RHIA, is a nationally recognized executive with progressive senior leadership experience in a wide range of healthcare organizations. As an RHIA, she has a successful track record in health information management, revenue cycle, risk management and quality improvement. Her MS in I-O Psychology, has fueled her passion about working with leaders to develop strategic thinking skills.

Christine Kalish, MBA, CMPE, is a senior executive and trusted healthcare advisor with deep experience in ambulatory care and academic medicine. She is a thought leader and strategist for emerging and expanding healthcare organizations. For more than thirty years, Kalish has been leading organizations and teams to develop critical infrastructure and growth planning to improve operations, workflow, human resources and revenue cycle. She continually searches for innovative ways to assist her clients so they can deliver quality care for the populations they serve.

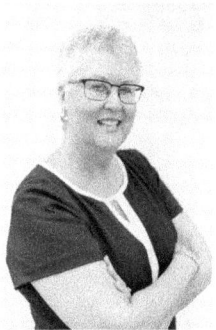

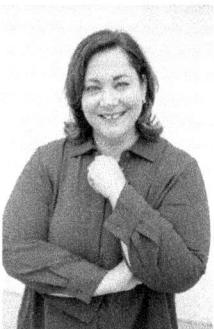

Sharon Z. Ginchansky, MAOM, is a consultant specializing in leadership and organizational change. Her career spans more than twenty-five years of operational and human resources experience working as an executive in the healthcare field.

Contributor: Summer Humphreys, MBA

www.ingramcontent.com/pod-product-compliance
Lightning Source LLC
Chambersburg PA
CBHW061304220326
41599CB00026B/4732